Expertise in the Operating Room

Michael Yaremchuk
Arman T. Serebrakian • Brent B. Pickrell
Julianna Paniss • Michael T. Bailin
Nicole Gangi
Editors

Expertise in the Operating Room

Logistics, Fundamentals and Nuances

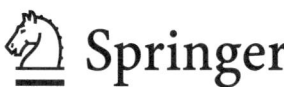

Editors
Michael Yaremchuk
Division of Plastic Surgery
Massachusetts General Hospital
Boston, MA, USA

Brent B. Pickrell
Department of Plastic Surgery
Harvard Medical School, Massachusetts
General Hospital
Boston, MA, USA

Michael T. Bailin
Department of Anesthesia
The Boston Center for Ambulatory Surgery
Boston, MA, USA

Arman T. Serebrakian
Division of Plastic Surgery
Harvard Medical School, Massachusetts
General Hospital
Boston, MA, USA

Julianna Paniss
The Boston Center for Ambulatory Surgery
Boston, MA, USA

Nicole Gangi
Department of Marketing
The Boston Center for Ambulatory Surgery
Boston, MA, USA

ISBN 978-3-031-30834-5   ISBN 978-3-031-30835-2 (eBook)
https://doi.org/10.1007/978-3-031-30835-2

© The Editor(s) (if applicable) and The Author(s), under exclusive license to Springer Nature Switzerland AG 2023

This work is subject to copyright. All rights are solely and exclusively licensed by the Publisher, whether the whole or part of the material is concerned, specifically the rights of translation, reprinting, reuse of illustrations, recitation, broadcasting, reproduction on microfilms or in any other physical way, and transmission or information storage and retrieval, electronic adaptation, computer software, or by similar or dissimilar methodology now known or hereafter developed.

The use of general descriptive names, registered names, trademarks, service marks, etc. in this publication does not imply, even in the absence of a specific statement, that such names are exempt from the relevant protective laws and regulations and therefore free for general use.

The publisher, the authors, and the editors are safe to assume that the advice and information in this book are believed to be true and accurate at the date of publication. Neither the publisher nor the authors or the editors give a warranty, expressed or implied, with respect to the material contained herein or for any errors or omissions that may have been made. The publisher remains neutral with regard to jurisdictional claims in published maps and institutional affiliations.

This Springer imprint is published by the registered company Springer Nature Switzerland AG
The registered company address is: Gewerbestrasse 11, 6330 Cham, Switzerland

To
Marilynn
Kait and Eliza
as well as
Charles and Deuce (Charles II)

Preface

A surgical operation is a detailed coordination of a complex procedure involving the integration of many people, facilities, and supplies. The efficiency and success of an operation foremost depends on the expertise of its staff. These medical professionals must understand their tasks and the operating room milieu.

The surgeon, surgeon's assistant, anesthesiologist, scrub nurse, and circulating and recovery room nurses all determine an operation's success and efficiency. Medical professional education too often focuses on senior level preparatory education or capstone projects rather than mastering the day-to-day practical information or techniques. A reflection of this quandary is the establishment of surgical intern "boot camps." These industry subsidized courses taken after medical school graduation are one- or two-week courses whose curriculum is to train recent graduates how to function as surgeons.

Patients deserve the work of professionals, not amateurs.

This book provides the logistics, fundamentals, and nuances for both the priests and the acolytes involved in surgery to coordinate and optimize performance and results in the operating room.

Boston, MA, USA	Michael Yaremchuk, MD
Boston, MA, USA	Arman T. Serebrakian, MD
Boston, MA, USA	Brent B. Pickrell, MD
Boston, MA, USA	Julianna Paniss
Boston, MA, USA	Michael T. Bailin, MD
Boston, MA, USA	Nicole Gangi

Acknowledgments

My coauthors, Residents in the Harvard Plastic Surgery Training Program and my colleagues at The Boston Center for Ambulatory Surgery, Inc. were indispensable in the preparation of this book.

Our illustrators Kip Carter and Ryoko Hamaguchi, MD, added artistic precision and nuance. Kip Carter is Chief of Medical Illustration Services at the College of Veterinary Medicine at the University of Georgia and Ryoko Hamaguchi, MD, is Plastic Surgery Resident at Harvard Mass General Brigham.

Nicole Gangi, Administrative Assistant and Marketing/Digital Marketing Specialist, painstakingly organized and coordinated this work.

Thank you all,
Dr. Y

Contents

Part I Preparation Before the Operating Room

1. **The Surgeon's Preparation Before the Operating Room** 3
   Michael Yaremchuk and David Straughan

2. **The Anesthesiologist's and Nursing Team's Preparation Before the Operating Room** 9
   Michael T. Bailin, Julianna Paniss, Polly-Ann Downey, and Michael Yaremchuk

Part II Preparation in the Operating Room-Before Anesthesia

3. **Universal Protocol** 23
   Polly-Ann Downey and Michael Yaremchuk

4. **Sterility** 27
   Julianna Paniss, Polly-Ann Downey, and Michael Yaremchuk

Part III Preparation in the Operating Room-After Anesthesia

5. **Patient Preparation** 35
   David Straughan, Polly-Ann Downey, Michael Yaremchuk, and Dylan Perry

Part IV Surgery

6. **Logistics and Ergonomics** 51
   David Straughan, Imran Ratanshi, Julianna Paniss, and Michael Yaremchuk

7. **Fire** 57
   David Mattos, Michael T. Bailin, and Michael Yaremchuk

Part V The Surgeon's Tools

8 Surgeon's Instruments 65
Eric J. Wenzinger, Timothy J. Irwin, and Michael Yaremchuk

9 Sutures and Needles 85
Brent B. Pickrell and Michael Yaremchuk

Part VI Surgical Devices

10 Local Anesthetics 103
Seth Fruge and Michael Yaremchuk

11 Electrocautery 111
Michael T. Bailin and Michael Yaremchuk

12 Surgical Tourniquets 121
David Mattos, Brent B. Pickrell, and Michael Yaremchuk

Part VII Wound Closure

13 Drains 129
Swapnil Kachare, David Straughan, and Michael Yaremchuk

14 Suture Closure 137
Brent B. Pickrell and Michael Yaremchuk

15 Surgical Dressings 149
Frankie Wong, Michael Yaremchuk, Lisa Gfrerer,
and Olivia Abbate Ford

Index 163

List of Videos

Video 4.1   Scrubbing
Video 4.2   Drying and gloving
Video 6.1   Suctioning
Video 8.1   Safely attaching and detaching a surgical blade from a knife handle
Video 9.1   Loading the needle driver
Video 12.1 Demonstration of proper upper extremity placement of a tourniquet
Video 14.1 One-handed knot tying
Video 14.2 Two-handed knot tying
Video 14.3 Continuous percutaneous closure
Video 14.4 Simple interrupted suture
Video 14.5 Vertical mattress suture
Video 14.6 Horizontal mattress suture

Contributors

Michael T. Bailin, MD Department of Anesthesia, The Boston Center for Ambulatory Surgery, Boston, MA, USA

Polly-Ann Downey, RN The Boston Center for Ambulatory Surgery, Inc., Boston, MA, USA

Olivia Abbate Ford, MD Harvard Plastic Surgery Residency Program, Boston, MA, USA

Seth Fruge, MD Harvard Mass General Brigham Plastic Surgery Residency Program, Boston, MA, USA

Nicole Gangi The Boston Center for Ambulatory Surgery, Boston, MA, USA

Lisa Gfrerer, MD, PhD Harvard Plastic Surgery Residency Program, Boston, MA, USA

Timothy J. Irwin, MD Harvard Mass General Brigham Plastic Surgery Residency Program, Boston, MA, USA

Swapnil Kachare, MD Massachusetts General Hospital and The Boston Center for Ambulatory Surgery, Inc., Boston, MA, USA

David Mattos, MD, MBA Harvard Mass General Brigham Plastic Surgery Residency Program, Boston, MA, USA

Julianna Paniss, CST The Boston Center for Ambulatory Surgery, Boston, MA, USA

Dylan Perry, MD Harvard Plastic Surgery Residency Program, Boston, MA, USA

Brent B. Pickrell, MD Harvard Mass General Brigham Plastic Surgery Residency Program, Boston, MA, USA

Imran Ratanshi, MD Division of Plastic Surgery, Massachusetts General Hospital and The Boston Center for Ambulatory Surgery, Inc., Boston, MA, USA

Arman T. Serebrakian, MD Harvard Mass General Brigham Plastic Surgery Residency Program, Boston, MA, USA

David Straughan, MD Division of Plastic Surgery, Massachusetts General Hospital and The Boston Center for Ambulatory Surgery, Inc., Boston, MA, USA

Eric J. Wenzinger, MD Harvard Mass General Brigham Plastic Surgery Residency Program, Boston, MA, USA

Frankie Wong, MD Harvard Mass General Brigham Plastic Surgery Residency Program, Boston, MA, USA

Michael Yaremchuk, MD Division of Plastic Surgery, Massachusetts General Hospital, Boston, MA, USA

The Boston Center for Ambulatory Surgery, Inc., Boston, MA, USA

Part I
Preparation Before the Operating Room

Chapter 1
The Surgeon's Preparation Before the Operating Room

Michael Yaremchuk and David Straughan

The surgeon bears fundamental responsibility to the patient for making an accurate diagnosis and planning the proper operation to solve the patient's problem. The scheduled operation dictates the actions of the rest of the operating team. The operation should be scheduled accurately, allowing staff to anticipate and plan appropriately for the procedure's duration, instrumentation, and postoperative care.

Responsibilities prior to entering the operating room for the surgeon and his team include the emotional and physical preparation of the patient. The patient must be educated about the goal and extent of surgery, its morbidity, and the anticipated recovery during preoperative consultation [1]. Appropriate education and preparation provide security in the patient's decision-making.

> *With this background, the patient's consent for surgery is ideally performed during the last preoperative consultation with the surgeon. Obtaining a consent on the morning of the operation by a delegate who is foreign to the patient is unlikely to create confidence and alleviate anxiety.*

A patient's surgical plan begins well before arriving at the preoperative setting. It is an important step to transition from "person" to "patient." Surgery-induced patient lifestyle changes are unique to each patient. The lifestyle changes should be anticipated by the caregivers and shared with the patient. Postsurgical-related schedules may impact child care, meal preparation, physical activity, and work. For

---

M. Yaremchuk (✉)
Division of Plastic Surgery, Massachusetts General Hospital, and The Boston Center for Ambulatory Surgery, Inc., Boston, MA, USA
e-mail: dr.y@dryaremchuk.com

D. Straughan
Massachusetts General Hospital and The Boston Center for Ambulatory Surgery, Inc., Boston, MA, USA

© The Author(s), under exclusive license to Springer Nature Switzerland AG 2023
M. Yaremchuk et al. (eds.), *Expertise in the Operating Room*, https://doi.org/10.1007/978-3-031-30835-2_1

those patients who have a serious medical illness, the primary medical team and specialists should be invited to participate in risk assessment and shared decision-making prior to surgery.

Preoperative surgical diagnosis should be focused not only on the patient's presenting complaint but also on their overall physical status relevant to the planned operation. A thorough patient evaluation will minimize the risk of surgical infection and systemic complications. Diabetes, smoking, and obesity all predispose a patient to infection and compromised wound healing. If appropriate, specialist consultations, laboratory, and radiologic measures should be done in a timely manner well ahead of the surgical date.

> *Additional data, if necessary, should be obtained with adequate time to allow medical compensatory actions. Data obtained on the day of surgery often result in operation day cancelation or compromised preparation.*

Preoperative preparations for the day of surgery include appropriate use and timing of personal medications; showering with soap or chlorhexidine the day prior to surgery; absence of makeup, lotion, deodorant, or other skin products; and removal of jewelry and piercings. See Appendix 1 "Preoperative Timeline" for an example of the preoperative instructions given to patients in anticipation of their planned surgery at The Boston Center for Ambulatory Surgery, Inc. Appendix 2 lists medications that alter coagulation. These should be avoided before the scheduled surgery.

Preoperative preparation also includes instructions for postoperative care and medications. For example, avoid inappropriate physical activity and medications, as well as smoking. Complications may or may not occur—most patients truly do not consider the scarring, bleeding, infections, and wound issues that occur with statistically unremitting constancy. Although they are critically concerned with the surgical and aesthetic outcome, there is no doubt that individuals want their experience to be a good one too.

Appendix 1: Patient Preoperative Timeline

Today

- STOP SMOKING. If you are a smoker, your planned surgery is an excellent impetus to stop. Smoking delays wound healing, which may compromise the result of your surgery. It also impairs your cardiovascular and respiratory systems. You should quit smoking as early as possible but at least 4–6 weeks prior to your planned surgery.
- Arrange to have any preoperative testing requested by your surgeon to be performed so that the results will be available 2 weeks prior to surgery. The attached prescription will inform your physician or hospital laboratory what tests are required. The results should be forwarded immediately to your plastic surgeon.

Two Weeks Before Surgery

- Stop taking aspirin- or ibuprofen-containing products for 2 weeks prior to surgery and 2 weeks following surgery. These products may cause bleeding. Many other products, such as Bufferin, Anacin, and Advil contain aspirin or ibuprofen. A list of aspirin- and ibuprofen-containing drugs that you must avoid is included. Tylenol (acetaminophen) may be used as a substitute.
- Avoid red wines for 2 weeks prior to surgery because they may give you a tendency to bleed and may increase bruising.
- As you will be sedated during surgery, it is necessary for you to have someone you know to pick you up from the surgery center or hospital. Unless you have made arrangements to spend the evening after surgery at the hospital or surgery center, it is important to have someone spend the first postoperative evening with you. Please make arrangements as we cannot discharge you without an escort.

Two Days Before Surgery

- Please call the surgeon's staff 2 days prior to surgery. Ask for the nurse to verify with you the preoperative instructions and confirm your arrival time for surgery.
- Be sure to ask the nurse if you should take or bring in your daily prescribed medications.
- Have post-op medications prescribed by your plastic surgeon filled by your pharmacist.

Day Before Surgery

- It is imperative that you have **NOTHING TO EAT OR DRINK AFTER MIDNIGHT THE EVENING BEFORE SURGERY** unless otherwise advised by your surgeon.
- Wash your hair with your usual shampoo the night before surgery.

Day of Surgery

- Take your usual prescription medications with a sip of water the morning of surgery. If you take insulin, discuss the appropriate dose with your surgeon preoperatively.

- Please report to the surgical facility on the day of surgery. Allow yourself ample travel time so that you arrive at the scheduled time for your surgery.
- Please leave all valuables and nonessential jewelry at home.
- **DO NOT WEAR ANY MAKEUP, FINGERNAIL POLISH, ARTIFICIAL FINGERNAILS, OR ARTIFICIAL EYELASHES** on the day of surgery as this will interfere with the surgery and cause delay.
- For your comfort, we suggest wearing shirts that button down the front and low-heeled, comfortable shoes. If you are having facial surgery, we advise you to bring a scarf and dark glasses.
- Bring reading glasses so that you can fill out forms. Do not wear contact lenses.
- You may shower the morning of surgery and wash your hair with your usual shampoo.

Appendix 2: Aspirin and Aspirin-Like Drugs to Avoid Before Surgery

To reduce your risk of bleeding during and after surgery, the following medicines should not be taken for at least 2 weeks prior to surgery.

This list is not all-inclusive; patients should look at the ingredients for medicines that contain aspirin or aspirin-like products.

4-Way cold tablets	Butalbital compound	Equagesic tablets	Motrin	Salflex tablets
Ache and pain tablets	Cama arthritis pain reliever	Equazine-M tablets	Nalfon	Salocol tablets
Acetycol	Cataflam tablets	Excedrin	Nalfon Pulvules	Salsitab
Actron	Children's Advil suspension	Feldene capsules	Naprosyn	Sk-65 compound caps
Adprin-B tablets	Children's Motrin suspension	Fiorgen PF tablets	Naproxen tablets	Sine-Off
Advil	Cheracol capsules	Fiorinal tablets	Nemugesic	Sine-Aid IB
Aggrenox	Cirin	Gensan	Nighttime effervescent	Sigmagen
Aleve	Clinoril	Goody's headache powder	Norgesic	Soma compound
Alka Seltzer	Congesprin	Halfprin tablets	Norgesic Forte	St. Joseph adult chewable aspirin
Alprin bi tablets	Cope tablets	Haltran tablets	Nuprin	Stendin
Amigesic	Coricidin	Histadyl	Nytol	Sulindac
Anacin	Convangesic	Ibu-Tab tablets	Orudis capsules	Supai
Anaprox	Daprisal	Ibuprofen	Oruvail capsules	Supac

Anaprox DS	Darvon compound	Indochron E-R capsules	Pabalate	Synalgos capsules
Anodynos	Darvo-Tran	Indocin	Pac tablets	Synalgos-DC capsules
Ansaid	Dasin	Indocin SR capsules	Pamprin-IB tablets	Talwin compound tablets
Argesic	Daypro	Indomethacin	Pentasa	Ticlid
Artha-G tablets	Decagesic	Ketoprofen capsules	Pentagesic	Tolectin
Arthritis Bayer timed release	Demerol CIAPC	Lanorinal tablets	Pepto-Bismol tablets and suspension	Toradol infection
Arthropan	Disalcid caps/tabs	Lodine	Percodan	Toradol tablets
Ascodeen-30	Doan's pills	Lovenox	Persantine	Trancogesic
Ascriptin	Dristan	Magan	Phenaphen	Trental
Asperbuf tablets	Duoprin-S syrup	Magnaprin arthritis strength	Piroxicam	Triaminicin
Aspergum	Duradyne	Magasal tablets	Plavix	Tricosal tablets
Aspirin	Duragesic	Maximum Bayer Aspirin	Ponstel capsules	Tri-pain tablets
Asirimox	Easprin	Meclomen (meclofenamate)	Predisal	Trigesic tablets
Bayer aspirin tablets	Ecotrin	Medaprin	Presalin	Trilisate tablets
BC tablet and powder	Edrisal	Menadol tablets	Pyrroxate	Trilisate liquid
Buf-tabs	Emagrin	Micrainin	Relafen	Vanquish
Buf-A comp	Empirin tablets	Midol	Robaxisal	Verin
Bufferin	Empiral	Mobidin	Rowasa	Voltaren tablets
Buffetts II tablets	Emprazil	Mobigesic	Rufen	Vitamin E
Buffex	Endodan	Monacet	S-A-C	Warfarin
Buffinol tablets	Epromate tablets	Monogesic	Saleto tablets	Zorprim tablets

Reference

1. Cole N. Informed consent: considerations in aesthetic and reconstructive surgery of the breast. Clin Plast Surg. 1988;15:541–8.

Chapter 2
The Anesthesiologist's and Nursing Team's Preparation Before the Operating Room

Michael T. Bailin, Julianna Paniss, Polly-Ann Downey, and Michael Yaremchuk

2.1 The Anesthesiologist

A successful surgical anesthetic should be measured or defined in terms of its outcome. Were the surgeon and patient satisfied? Specifically, the surgeon requires "good operating conditions," and that may mean anything from an awake patient providing verbal feedback during a brain biopsy to an unconscious, intubated individual with deep neuromuscular blockade for abdominal surgery. Ensuring stable vital signs throughout the procedure rounds out the definition of a competent anesthetic. Most patients expect to have no memory and no discomfort during the procedure.

Anesthesiologists participate in a preoperative review to elucidate underlying significant medical conditions, factor in the planned surgical goals, and, in this manner, ensure a custom anesthetic strategy to achieve a safe and effective outcome.

M. T. Bailin
Department of Anesthesia, The Boston Center for Ambulatory Surgery, Boston, MA, USA

J. Paniss · P.-A. Downey
The Boston Center for Ambulatory Surgery, Inc., Boston, MA, USA

M. Yaremchuk (✉)
Division of Plastic Surgery, Massachusetts General Hospital, and The Boston Center for Ambulatory Surgery, Inc., Boston, MA, USA
e-mail: dr.y@dryaremchuk.com

© The Author(s), under exclusive license to Springer Nature Switzerland AG 2023
M. Yaremchuk et al. (eds.), *Expertise in the Operating Room*,
https://doi.org/10.1007/978-3-031-30835-2_2

Evidence-based, data-driven pathways for preoperative assessment and workup indicate which tests have value and should be performed. These algorithms have shown that chest radiographs, electrocardiograms (ECGs), electrolytes, and coagulation testing are not necessary prior to ambulatory elective surgery in the vast majority of patients.

Specific testing guidelines have been widely published, and the American Society of Anesthesiology last updated its recommendations in 2012 [1].

Even when some abnormalities are identified (e.g., hypertension in the pre-op holding area or hypokalemia in a patient on diuretics), anesthesiologists are increasingly likely to proceed with surgery when there is scant evidence to suggest postponement in the hope that "optimizing" a specific variable will improve morbidty, mortality, or decrease complications. Although we all want our patients to be in the best shape possible prior to surgery, this optimization occurs under the care and guidance of the primary care provider prior to planned elective surgery.

There is a "risk management" element to proceeding with surgery with the presence of abnormalities, and the anesthesiologist should specifically comment on any anomaly in their preoperative workup. Even patients admitting to cocaine use in the 48 h prior to surgery have not demonstrated to have worse outcomes if they present with normal vital signs and demonstrate no electrocardiographic ectopy [2, 3].

Red flag diagnoses, such as unstable angina, recent congestive heart failure, or pneumonia, must be identified as the risks of major adverse cardiac and pulmonary events increase substantially (Table 2.1) [4, 5].

A thorough preoperative assessment performed by the procedural team will generally reveal that the patient is ready and appropriately prepared for anesthesia and surgery. Distinct attention should be paid if a patient presents with evidence of a condition where special precaution and further investigation may improve the surgical outcome. Using guidelines published by the American College of Cardiology and the American Heart Association, most plastic and reconstructive surgery and office-based procedures are at the low end of the risk spectrum. Examples of common diagnoses or historical findings that may alter patient management are in the "red flag" table.

2.1.1 Patient History, Physical Exam, and Laboratory Assessment

The standard of care requires a member of the anesthesia care team to perform a history and physical examination appropriate for the proposed surgery.

Obtaining and reviewing old anesthesia records is most advantageous when a patient reports a previous problem with anesthesia.

An excellent practice is to review each patient's chart on a day prior to surgery, with attention to the specific history supplied by the patient.

Table 2.1 Cardiac and pulmonary red flag diagnoses [5–10]

Red flag	Issue	Rationale/background	Actions
Opioid use disorder (OUD)	Opioid use may increase tolerance. IV opioid injection is associated with serious infectious diseases, including hepatitis, endocarditis, and HIV	Withdrawal symptoms may occur post-op. Usual doses of opioids may be ineffective	Patients with substance use disorder are poor candidates for elective surgery and should be referred to a specialized clinic for treatment
Cocaine intoxication	Acute administration may cause coronary vasospasm and precipitate myocardial ischemia, myocardial infarction, ventricular dysrhythmia, hypertension, and tachycardia	Cocaine is an indirectly acting sympathomimetic amine that blocks the presynaptic uptake of norepinephrine and dopamine, increasing synaptic transmission	At present, there is no consensus on the timing of cocaine abstinence prior to elective surgery. Case reports suggest that 8 h is sufficient for general anesthesia if the patient is stable. Consider waiting for 24 h in an outpatient setting. Limit or avoid local anesthetics containing epinephrine
Beta-blockers	Beta-blockers should generally be continued on the day of surgery	Abrupt withdrawal of beta-blockade may result in ischemia or myocardial infarction	Assess the home medication list and administer p.o. or IV beta-blockade in the perioperative period
ACE and ARB	Persistent and profound hypotension may occur after the induction of anesthesia in patients taking renin-angiotensin system inhibitors	Angiotensin-converting enzyme inhibitors (ACEI) and angiotensin receptor blockers (ARB) are often associated with potent vasodilatory events after anesthesia induction	Discontinuation of renin-angiotensin system inhibitors 24 h prior to elective surgery may mitigate severe postinduction hypotension. Vasopressin or norepinephrine should be available to treat refractory vasodilatory shock
Anticoagulants	Long-acting antiplatelet or antithrombotic agents are prescribed for multiple medical conditions and may increase perioperative bleeding if continued during surgery	Specific consideration of clinical indications and management strategy must be addressed before advising discontinuation	The decision to administer or omit antiplatelet or anticoagulant should be based on the risk of surgical bleeding and discussion with the prescribing provider. The appropriate interval for omitting anticoagulation should be decided uniquely for each patient

(continued)

Table 2.1 (continued)

Red flag	Issue	Rationale/background	Actions
Hx or family history of venous thrombosis	Determine what VTE prophylaxis is most suitable, depending on each individual patient's risk factors for postoperative DVT	Patients with several risk factors may benefit from pharmaceutical-based prophylaxis regimens	Assess risk using the VTE risk assessment scale. Example at https://www.med.umich.edu/clinical/images/VTE-Risk-Assessment.pdf Example: 70 y.o. obese female with a history of DVT is at high risk for new VTE
Addiction treatment	Buprenorphine or naltrexone taken for OUD may interfere with effective postoperative pain management. Tolerance to opioids (including methadone) may result in excessive doses, which can cause respiratory depression	Opioid agonists are blocked at the opioid receptor by buprenorphine and naltrexone. The typical opioid narcotic dosage used for postoperative pain may be inadequate due to tolerance to the agonist or a receptor blockade	Preoperative counseling should set expectations regarding pain management, especially in patients with preexisting chronic pain. Provide local anesthesia and consider additional long-acting local anesthetics for post-op pain. Add appropriate narcotics and analgesics (including NSAIDS) for postoperative pain control The pain or addiction specialist should be available for assistance during postoperative management. It is appropriate to continue the prescribed dosages of methadone on the day of surgery
Recent percutaneous coronary intervention (PCI)	Specific recommendations exist for postponing elective surgery after recent PCI, such as angioplasty and stent placement	The risks of stent thrombosis and surgical hemorrhage must be taken into account prior to scheduling nonurgent invasive procedures	Cardiology consultation is mandatory. Based on expert opinion and published guidelines, a patient-specific written note will guide the surgical team on medical management and the timing for elective surgery
Heart rate abnormality	Newly irregular heart rate, profound bradycardia, or unexpected tachycardia	Rapid heart rates are often attributed to anxiety but may indicate cardiovascular instability. Underlying pathology should be ruled out	Consider medical consultation and delay of surgery if HR <40 or >120 or if there is a new arrhythmia
Blood pressure abnormality	Unexpected systolic or diastolic hypertension that does not promptly normalize after initial readings prior to surgery	BP can be expected to increase even further post-op, secondary to pain, additional fluid, and interruption of antihypertensive medications	Consider medical consultation and delay of surgery if systolic BP remains >180 mmHg and/or diastolic BP remains >100 mmHg

New cough	Potential upper or lower respiratory infection, COVID-19, bronchitis, reactive airway disease, or acid reflux	An acute change in respiratory status may indicate inflammation and increased risks of atelectasis, pneumonia, and abnormal gas exchange	Coughing and pulmonary secretions may worsen postoperatively due to the progression of airway disease and general anesthesia. Increased arterial and venous pressure from excessive coughing may promote hematoma formation and wound dehiscence
Morbid obesity	Patients may have undiagnosed pulmonary hypertension. Right ventricular strain and hypoxemia worsened with respiratory depression. Increased risk for atelectasis and difficult airway management	Patients with a body mass index >40 are at a greater risk for obstructive sleep apnea (OSA). Obese patients are also at a greater risk for wound infections, blood clots, and pneumonia	Screen patients for OSA; bring a CPAP device on the day of surgery; consider overnight admission Screening tools (e.g., STOP-BANG questionnaire) may help identify patients at risk and stratify risk management
Diagnosis of obstructive sleep apnea (OSA) or pre-op screen suggesting OSA	Cardiovascular, pulmonary, and metabolic pathophysiology accompanying OSA, whether due to obesity or other causes, increases the risk for difficult airway management	Greater risk of desaturation and airway compromise Untreated OSA puts patients at a higher risk for post-op hypoxemia	Refer patients for polysomnograms if a diagnosis is suspected but not confirmed Bring a CPAP device for post-op respiratory support Have additional airway equipment Consider surgery in an inpatient setting
History or physical examination consistent with difficult airway	Difficult mask ventilation and endotracheal intubation are associated with hypoxemia and respiratory arrest	The risks of pharyngeal collapse, inability to ventilate or oxygenate, and respiratory compromise are higher in morbid obesity	If airway examination reveals a short neck, large tongue, small mouth, large tonsils, and/or excessive palatal soft tissues, specialized equipment should be ready prior to the induction of anesthesia. Limit or omit opioid use
Gastroesophageal reflux	Risks of vocal cord irritation, coughing, bronchospasm, and aspiration are increased	Gastric contents may reflux into the esophagus and pharynx with acidic secretions entering the airway. Obesity, pregnancy, and diabetes increase aspiration risk	Treat with H2 antagonists and proton-pump inhibitors on the day of surgery. The PPI should also be administered orally the night before the procedure in severe cases Confirm NPO and fasting intervals preoperatively. Consider gastrokinetic agents such as metoclopramide

Using a standard form ensures completeness in the recording of relevant historical items and issues of medical significance.

2.1.1.1 Anesthesia-Specific History Form

- *Are there recent changes in your medical history? (A recent upper respiratory tract infection (URI) may lead to more coughing and respiratory complications after general anesthesia.)*
- *Do you have sleep apnea or use continuous positive airway pressure (CPAP)? (This may alter how opioids are prescribed after surgery.)*
- *What medicines do you take? (You can give specific instructions on what to take/omit prior to the day of surgery—especially for blood pressure, anticoagulation, and diabetes management.)*
- *Do you have a pacemaker or other implanted electrical device? (Learn more about the device.)*
- *Do you have metallic body piercings?*
- *What previous surgery have you had?*
- *Were there any problems with the anesthesia?*
- *Do you take painkillers daily?*
- *Do you take suboxone or methadone?*
- *For female patients: Is there any possibility you may be pregnant?*
- *Do you have gastric (acid) reflux symptoms?*

Patients who take prescription medicine for cardiac disease (antianginals, anticoagulants, beta-blockers), or other serious medical conditions, deserve custom guidance and clear-cut instructions on what to take and what medications to omit on the day before and the day of surgery, particularly if they are receiving general anesthesia.

For example, patients who take their regular dose of an angiotensin receptor blocker (e.g., losartan, valsartan) or an angiotensin-converting enzyme inhibitor (e.g., lisinopril, captopril) on the day of surgery are much more likely to have severe hypotension requiring vasopressor support and other complications.

Ideally, patients are asked for these data as part of the surgical consultation. When surgery is scheduled, registered nurses or surgical office staff would be responsible to coordinate the flow of critical information to the appropriate members of the team. Effective teamwork in surgical practice will positively affect safety, patient experience, and overall outcome.

2.1.1.2 Patient Physical Examination

The anesthesia provider will focus their physical exam on the airway and vital signs. The assessment of height and weight helps establish initial drug doses and the sizes of airway equipment to be prepared. The standard of care mandates that "immediate preinduction" blood pressure, oxygen saturation, and heart rate and rhythm be ***measured and recorded*** prior to the induction of anesthesia.

The relevant physical examinations will include an examination of the mouth opening, the presence of dentures, and missing or capped teeth and a gross examination of the neck and trachea. The presence of wheezing, rales, or rhonchi as well as abnormal heart sounds should be noted. Patients who are elderly or have known cardiopulmonary disease, adventitious lung sounds, carotid bruits, or cardiac murmurs may indicate new or actionable pathophysiology.

As the data from the history, physical exam, and chart review are compiled, the decision can be made whether to perform the surgery in a same-day surgical unit versus a hospital or to admit the patient (e.g., the patient on suboxone for pain control, the severely obese for respiratory monitoring). Even patients with several comorbidities, provided they are appropriately screened and medically well managed by their primary team, will routinely have excellent outcomes after anesthesia and surgery in outpatient settings.

2.1.1.3 Cardiac Risk Assessment

2.1.1.3.1 METs and Perioperative Risk

Metabolic equivalents (METs) are based on activities of daily living, such as walking, running, and other activity.

In general, patients who have cardiac history, but remain asymptomatic and stable, and can perform activities at 4 METs or greater are considered to have good functional capacity.

They are at low risk for adverse cardiac events following superficial, plastic, and reconstructive surgery.

2.1.1.3.2 Examples of Activities Greater Than 4 METs

– Walking at 4 mph
– Running a short distance
– Doing yard work (raking or mowing)
– Recreational sports (golf, tennis, and swimming)

2.1.1.3.3 Examples of Activities Less Than 4 METs

– Walking indoors around the house
– Walking one to two blocks on a level ground
– Walking outside at 2–3 mph
– Light household work (doing dishes)
– Personal care (dressing, eating, or bathing)

As the data from the history, physical exam, and chart review are compiled, the decision can be made whether to perform the surgery in a same-day surgical unit versus at a hospital or to admit the patient (e.g., the patient on suboxone for pain control, the severely obese for respiratory monitoring). Even patients with several comorbidities, provided they are appropriately screened and medically well managed by their primary team, will routinely have excellent outcomes after anesthesia and surgery in outpatient settings.

2.1.2 Surgical and Cardiac Risk Assessment

Three surgical risk calculators are in common use. These are useful interactive tools for assessing risks for perioperative morbidity and mortality.

Gupta Calculator: https://qxmd.com/calculate/calculator_245/gupta-perioperative-cardiac-risk
NSQIP Calculator: https://riskcalculator.facs.org/RiskCalculator/
RCRI Calculator: https://www.mdcalc.com/revised-cardiac-risk-index-pre-operative-risk

In general, proceed with elective surgery if the cardiac risk is <1% and the patient can perform >4 METS activity. Consider elective surgery carefully if the cardiac risk is >1% and METS <4 or there is a new arrhythmia or ECG change.

Avoid elective surgery in the presence of the following:

- Active or recent acute coronary syndrome
- Percutaneous coronary intervention in the last 6 months
- Stroke in the last 3 months
- Venous thromboembolism in the last 3 months

(Reference [1, 5])

2.1.2.1 Airway Assessment

A careful history and physical examination will identify important factors regarding airway management and the potential for encountering difficulty.

Disease states or medical conditions with implications for airway management and patency include the following:

- Anatomical factors: small mandible with a receding chin, large tongue, small mouth opening, prominent upper incisors, or thyromental distance
- Congenital maxillofacial deformity
- Arthritis: reduced temporomandibular joint (TMJ) and/or neck mobility
- Obesity: excess soft tissue impairing laryngoscopy or postoperative obstruction

- Trauma: limited mouth opening or burn contracture
- History: difficult intubation, treatment for sleep apnea, or gastric reflux

2.2 Appropriate Anesthetic Materials

2.2.1 Standard Preparation

- Anesthesia machine/safety checkout before the case begins, gas tanks, scavenging, intravenous fluids (IVs), warmer, suction, nasogastric (NG) tube, and infusion pump
- Stethoscope, tubes, supraglottic airways, oropharyngeal airway (OPA)/ nasopharyngeal airway (NPA), stylet, and video laryngoscope
- Cognitive aid (the Stanford Manual)

2.2.2 Emergency Equipment/Planning for Crisis/Contingency

- Know how to call for help.
- Do drills with the team (code/laryngospasm/anaphylaxis/local anesthesia toxicity).
- Defibrillator and pacer.
- Backup positive pressure (self-inflating bag/Ambu).
- Cricothyrotomy kit.

2.2.3 Appropriate Medications

Ten to fifteen distinct drugs are administered to an individual patient in a typical anesthetic for surgery. A list would likely include one or more opioids (e.g., fentanyl/dilaudid), antibiotics (commonly cefazolin), multiple antiemetics, muscle relaxants, local anesthetics, general anesthetics, and reversal agents. Differentiating a true immune response (allergy) from a side effect or adverse drug reaction during surgery is essential.

2.2.3.1 Routine

Propofol, lidocaine, opioids, benzodiazepines, antiemetics, nonsteroidal anti-inflammatory drugs (NSAIDs), vasopressors, beta-blockers, neuromuscular blockers, ketamine, etomidate

2.2.3.2 Emergency

Dantrolene, intralipid, inotropes, epinephrine, adenosine.

2.3 Possible Need for Transfusion

Although the risk that a blood transfusion will result in adverse complications is very low, the surgeon and anesthesiologist should assess the potential for bleeding preoperatively. A careful review of the patient's medical history should focus on anemia and medications that may affect hemostasis.

> In general, a reasonably healthy patient can shed 1000–1200 cc of blood and will not require a blood transfusion, provided euvolemia is maintained with an intravenous balanced salt solution.

Risks associated with transfusing blood remain quite low. Clinical trials have shown that restrictive transfusion practices are associated with better long-term outcomes than liberal transfusion.

> In a euvolemic patient, hemoglobin of 7 gm/100 cc blood (generally equivalent to a patient with a hematocrit of 21%) is well tolerated.
> As an example, a patient with a hematocrit of 36 (or better) will be able to lose one third of their blood volume and have a final hematocrit of approximately 24% or a Hgb of 8 gm/100 dL.
> A patient weighing 150 lb has a total blood volume of approximately 4 L. This means they can tolerate losing 1300 cc of blood, which is equivalent to losing (or donating) three units of blood.

2.4 Perioperative/Circulator Nurse

The perioperative nurse/circulator provides continuity of care designed to meet individual patient needs through collaboration with other members of the operative team. The nurse reviews the scheduled operative procedures and patient history to address relevant patient issues—for example, sensory and motor deficits, anxiety, and obesity. The nursing team secures personal belongings, describes the pre- and postoperative patient experience, and provides appropriate patient clothing for the operating room.

On patient arrival, outside of the operating room (OR), the circulating nurse confirms the patient's identity, surgical expectation, operative site, and nil per os (NPO) status as well as records temperature and vital signs. Before escorting the patient into the OR, the circulating nurse confirms whether the consents are signed. The circulating nurse must have the necessities for surgery prepared in advance—operating room table, suction and cautery equipment, materials for patient preparation, and relevant X-rays. The nursing team is responsible for the availability of patient records with laboratory values and radiologic studies.

2.5 Scrub Nurse/Scrub Technologist

Understanding the surgical procedure is key to anticipating the needs for the operation.

A discussion with the surgeon prior to setting up the operating room will assure intraoperative access to all equipment pertinent to the operation, such as sutures, instruments, and devices. Surgeon preference cards will list all other materials required for the surgery. It is critical to have all necessary equipment prior to the patient being in the operating room to prevent any unnecessary complications or delays.

References

1. Arnett DK, Blumenthal RS, Albert MA, et al. 2019 ACC/AHA guideline on the primary prevention of cardiovascular disease: a report of the ACC/AHA task force on clinical practice guidelines. J Am Coll Cardiol. 2019.
2. Committee on Standards and Practice Parameters, Apfelbaum JL, Connis RT, Nickinovich DG, American Society of Anesthesiologists Task Force on Preanesthesia Evaluation, Pasternak LR, Arens JF, Caplan RA, Connis RT, Fleisher LA, Flowerdew R, Gold BS, Mayhew JF, Nickinovich DG, Rice LJ, Roizen MF, Twersky RS. Practice advisory for preanesthesia evaluation: an updated report by the American Society of Anesthesiologists Task Force on Preanesthesia Evaluation. Anesthesiology. 2012;116(3):522–38. https://doi.org/10.1097/ALN.0b013e31823c1067. PMID: 22273990.
3. Moon TS, Gonzales MX, Sun JJ, Kim A, Fox PE, Minhajuddin AT, Pak TJ, Ogunnaike B. Recent cocaine use and the incidence of hemodynamic events during general anesthesia: a retrospective cohort study. J Clin Anesth. 2019;55:146–50. https://doi.org/10.1016/j.jclinane.2018.12.028. Epub 2019 Jan 16. PMID: 30660093.
4. Matei V, Sami Haddadin A. Systemic and pulmonary arterial hypertension. In: Hines RL, Marschall KE, editors. Stoelting's anesthesia and co-existing disease. 6th ed. Philadelphia: Elsevier Saunders; 2012. p. 104–19.
5. Fleisher LA, Beckman JA, Brown KA, et al. ACC/AHA 2007 guidelines on perioperative cardiovascular evaluation and care for noncardiac surgery: a report of the American College of Cardiology/American Heart Association task force on practice guidelines (writing committee to revise the 2002 guidelines on perioperative cardiovascular evaluation for noncardiac surgery): developed in collaboration with the American Society of Echocardiography, American Society of Nuclear Cardiology, Heart Rhythm Society, Society of Cardiovascular Anesthesiologists, Society for Cardiovascular Angiography and Interventions, Society for Vascular Medicine and Biology, and Society for Vascular Surgery. Circulation. 2007;116(17):e418–99.
6. Al-Ruzzeh S, Kurup V. Respiratory diseases. In: Hines RL, Marschall KE, editors. Stoelting's anesthesia and coexisting disease. 6th ed. Philadelphia: Elsevier Saunders; 2012. p. 181–217.
7. Joshi GP, Ankichetty SP, Gan TJ, et al. Special article: society for ambulatory anesthesia consensus statement on preoperative selection of adult patients with obstructive sleep apnea scheduled for ambulatory surgery. Anesth Analg. 2012;115(5):1060–8. Anesthetic Management of Common Illnesses 435.
8. Ankichetty S, Chung F. Considerations for patients with obstructive sleep apnea undergoing ambulatory surgery. Curr Opin Anaesthesiol. 2011;24(6):605–11.
9. Ng A, Smith G. Gastroesophageal reflux and aspiration of gastric contents in anesthetic practice. Anesth Analg. 2001;93(2):494–513.
10. Granite EL, Farber NJ, Adler P. Parameters for treatment of cocaine-positive patients. J Oral Maxillofac Surg. 2007;65(10):1984–9.

Part II
Preparation in the Operating Room-Before Anesthesia

Chapter 3
Universal Protocol

Polly-Ann Downey and Michael Yaremchuk

3.1 Universal Protocol

The "Universal Protocol" is a checklist a surgeon must go through with their surgical team before beginning to operate [1]. The three steps a surgeon must follow before beginning a procedure are listed below.

3.1.1 Conduct a Preprocedure Verification Process

The surgeon, along with all healthcare professionals present during the procedure, must address missing information or discrepancies before starting. This process includes verification of the correct surgery and site, as well as verifying the signed patient consent form.

P.-A. Downey
The Boston Center for Ambulatory Surgery, Inc., Boston, MA, USA

M. Yaremchuk (✉)
Division of Plastic Surgery, Massachusetts General Hospital, and The Boston Center for Ambulatory Surgery, Inc., Boston, MA, USA
e-mail: dr.y@dryaremchuk.com

© The Author(s), under exclusive license to Springer Nature Switzerland AG 2023
M. Yaremchuk et al. (eds.), *Expertise in the Operating Room*, https://doi.org/10.1007/978-3-031-30835-2_3

3.1.2 Mark the Procedure Site

The protocol requires that at the minimum, the surgeon must mark the surgical site when there is more than one possible location for the procedure. The surgeon should clearly label the area where the surgery should be performed with a surgical marker. The surgeon should mark the line the incision should follow as well as the word "yes."

3.1.3 Perform a Time-Out

A time-out must be performed prior to the first incision or procedure starting. During the time-out, everything in the operating room is to come to a stop. All movements and conversations must be paused. The circulating nurse or designated member of the surgical team states the patient's name, their date of birth, the surgery to be performed as noted on the signed patient consent form, all patient allergies, and preoperative antibiotic administration. At the conclusion of the time-out, a fire risk assessment is done. Fire risks that are evaluated prior to surgery include the following: whether the incision is made above the xiphoid process, the use of cautery or a light source, the use of open oxygen, and the use of alcohol prep.

All participating members of the surgical team should be present during the time-out, and the procedure cannot begin until all questions and concerns are resolved. The team must verbally agree that the patient is the correct patient, that the correct procedure is going to be carried out, and that the surgery is going to be performed at the correct site. The time-out represents the final recapitulation and reassurance of accurate patient identity, surgical site, and procedure.

Appendix

Speak Up™

The Universal Protocol for Preventing Wrong Site, Wrong Procedure, and Wrong Person Surgery™

Guidance for Healthcare Professionals

Conduct a Preprocedure Verification Process

Address missing information or discrepancies before starting the procedure.

- Verify the correct procedure for the correct patient at the correct site.
- When possible, involve the patient in the verification process.

- Identify the items that must be available for the procedure.
- Use a standardized list to verify the availability of items for the procedure. (It is not necessary to document that the list was used for each patient.) At a minimum, these items include the following:
  - Relevant documentation (examples: history and physical, signed consent form, preanesthesia assessment)
  - Labeled diagnostic and radiology test results that are properly displayed (examples: radiology images and scans, pathology reports, biopsy reports)
  - Any required blood products, implants, devices, and special equipment
- Match the items that are to be available in the procedure area to the patient.

Mark the Procedure Site

At a minimum, mark the site when there is more than one possible location for the procedure and when performing the procedure in a different location could harm the patient.

- For spinal procedures: Mark the general spinal region on the skin. Special intraoperative imaging techniques may be used to locate and mark the exact vertebral level.
- Mark the site before the procedure is performed.
- If possible, involve the patient in the site-marking process.
- The site is marked by a licensed independent practitioner who is ultimately accountable for the procedure and will be present when the procedure is performed.
- In limited circumstances, site marking may be delegated to some medical residents, physician assistants (PAs), or advanced practice registered nurses (APRNs).
- Ultimately, the licensed independent practitioner is accountable for the procedure –even when delegating site marking.
- The mark is unambiguous and is used consistently throughout the organization.
- The mark is made at or near the procedure site.
- The mark is sufficiently permanent to be visible after skin preparation and draping.
- Adhesive markers are not the sole means of marking the site.
- For patients who refuse site marking or when it is technically or anatomically impossible or impractical to mark the site (see examples below): Use your organization's written, alternative process to ensure that the correct site is operated on. Examples of situations that involve alternative processes are as follows:
  - Mucosal surfaces or perineum
  - Minimal access procedures treating a lateralized internal organ, whether percutaneous or through a natural orifice
  - Teeth
  - Premature infants, for whom the mark may cause a permanent tattoo

Perform a Time-Out

The procedure is not started until all questions or concerns are resolved.

- Conduct a time-out immediately before starting the invasive procedure or making the incision.
- A designated member of the team starts the time-out.
- The time-out is standardized.
- The time-out involves the immediate members of the procedure team: the individual performing the procedure, anesthesia providers, a circulating nurse, an operating room technician, and other active participants who will be participating in the procedure from the beginning.
- All relevant members of the procedure team actively communicate during the time-out.
- During the time-out, the team members agree, at a minimum, on the following:
  - Correct patient identity
  - Correct site
  - Procedure to be done
- When the same patient has two or more procedures: If the person performing the procedure changes, another time-out needs to be performed before starting each procedure.
- Document the completion of the time-out. The organization determines the amount and type of documentation.

This document has been adapted from the full Universal Protocol. For specific requirements of the Universal Protocol, see The Joint Commission Standards.

Reference

1. The Joint Commission. Speakup: the universal protocol—The Joint Commission. https://www.jointcommission.org/-/media/tjc/documents/standards/universal-protocol/up_poster1pdf.pdf

Chapter 4
Sterility

Julianna Paniss, Polly-Ann Downey, and Michael Yaremchuk

4.1 The Operating Staff

4.1.1 Attire: Clothing, Headwear, Jewelry, and Footwear

Proper operating room (OR) attire is critical to help reduce surgical field contamination. This includes gowns (scrubs), footwear, and headwear. Scrubs must be worn in the operating room and perioperative areas. Scrubs should not be worn outside of the operating room. A cleaned scrub set should be changed daily or after contamination during the operative day. Footwear should be clean and dedicated to operating room use only. Outside footwear should be covered appropriately with disposable shoe covers or dedicated solely to use in the OR. All facial hair, including beards, should be covered with surgical head dressings. Linen surgical caps should be laundered daily and not worn outside of the OR. Single-use caps and bouffants should be discarded at the end of the operating day or when exiting the perioperative areas.

Supplementary Information The online version contains supplementary material available at https://doi.org/10.1007/978-3-031-30835-2_4.

J. Paniss · P.-A. Downey
The Boston Center for Ambulatory Surgery, Inc., Boston, MA, USA

M. Yaremchuk (✉)
Division of Plastic Surgery, Massachusetts General Hospital, and The Boston Center for Ambulatory Surgery, Inc., Boston, MA, USA
e-mail: dr.y@dryaremchuk.com

Masks must be worn when in the operating room if surgery is in progress or if any sterile instruments are exposed. Jewelry should not be worn during surgical procedures and their preparation.

The appropriate use of OR attire has become lax over the last few decades. When the senior author was being trained as a doctor in the 1970s and 1980s, they were forbidden to leave the hospital in scrubs. Medical professionals changed into OR attire upon entering the hospital and changed out of their attire before leaving the hospital to reduce the risk of transferring potentially contaminated environmental pathogens. Whereas it was previously verboten, it is not uncommon now to see staff wearing their OR attire outside of the OR, such as in lunchrooms, and also outside of the hospital, such as on public transportation, in stores, or while at play. *It is not hard to associate this lax behavior with the abundance of nosocomial infections present today.*

4.1.2 Hand Preparation: "Scrubbing"

Prior to patient or equipment preparation, the surgeon should scrub their hands.
General principles include the following:

1. Keep the fingernails short. Remove debris from underneath the fingernails. Do not wear false or long fingernails when scrubbing.
2. Visualize anatomic parts (fingers, hand, forearm) as four-sided objects. Focus on scrubbing each surface.
3. Scrub from distal to proximal, from fingertips to the proximal forearm.
4. Ensure water runs from distal to proximal so that water cannot make contact with unprepped areas around the elbow and then drip down onto the hands.

Traditionally, surgical scrubbing with medicated soap has been the gold standard to reduce the bacterial colonization of the surgeon's skin and is a time-honored ritual for preparation for surgery. Recent data have suggested that high-concentration alcohol-based formulations may have faster and longer-lasting bacterial decolonization effects than scrubbing with medicated soap and water. There are many formulations of hand preparation [1–4]. Most are similar to the skin prep agents described below and contain povidone-iodine, chlorhexidine, alcohol, para-chloro-meta-xylenol, or some mixture. There is no clear consensus between medicated soap and water versus alcohol-based foams or gels, so institutional guidelines take precedence and dictate practice. Some institutions favor a policy of a medicated surgical scrub for the first day's operation, requesting an alcohol-based formulation for subsequent operations.

4.1.3 Avoiding Hand Contamination: "Scrubbed" Hand Position

To avoid scrubbed hands becoming contaminated from unprepped areas above the elbow, the medical professional should enter the operating room with arms outstretched and hands maintained above the waist (see Video 4.1).

4.1.4 Hand Drying

After receiving a sterile towel from the scrub nurse or scrub technologist, dry both hands from distal to proximal, avoiding contact between the hands and the nonsterile surfaces. One side of the towel should be used for each arm. Avoid reusing any area of the towel. After the towel is discarded, the scrub nurse/scrub technologist will don the professional's surgical gown by holding it to allow the surgeon to place outstretched hands through the sleeves. The circulator nurse, who remains unsterile, will then secure the posterior part of the gown. To glove, the surgeon's right hand is brought through the wrist cuff of the right sleeve first (to the level of the proximal hand, allowing all digits and thumb to be exposed) and then placed directly into the glove with the scrub nurse/scrub technologist's assistance. The process is repeated on the left. A second pair of gloves may be worn for an additional layer of sterility and for the surgeon's own protection (see Video 4.2).

4.1.5 OR Environment

OR traffic should be limited. Visitors should adhere to the same behavior and attire as the operating room staff. The surgeon or scrub nurse/scrub technologist should be immediately notified of observed breaks in the sterile technique so that the problem can be rectified immediately.

4.1.6 Instruments

The sterilization of surgical instruments is paramount for safe surgery. Most surgical instruments are stainless steel and designed for reuse after they have been properly cleaned, disinfected, and sterilized. Some instruments are not steel or have intricate machinery or lenses, making them more complex to sterilize.

After use in an operation, instruments are first cleansed, whereby foreign material is removed with water and detergents. Cleansing can be performed by hand or with automated machines, depending on the complexity and fragility of the instrument. The instruments are then disinfected with a liquid that kills microorganisms (viruses and bacteria). Most disinfectants cannot kill spores (dormant bacteria that are not replicating and are more resistant to adverse chemicals in their environment). Finally, the instruments are sterilized. The gold standard sterilization technique is with high heat (and pressure), typically with steam in an autoclave machine. A full sterilization cycle for wrapped instruments will require a 30-min exposure time at 121 °C and then 15 min at 132 °C and a 15–30-min dry time. Autoclave treatment inactivates all fungi, bacteria, viruses, and bacterial spores. Some instruments that cannot be sterilized are only disinfected.

Flash sterilization or "immediate use steam sterilization" is considered an acceptable method for processing cleaned patient-care items that are able to be packaged, sterilized, and stored before use. The traditional flash cycle is 3-min exposure at 270–275 °F for nonporous items and 10-min exposure at 270–275 °F for porous items.

(A comprehensive discussion of this topic is available through the Centers for Disease Control and Prevention (https://www.cdc.gov/infectioncontrol/guidelines/disinfection/index.html).)

4.2 Patient

4.2.1 Preoperative Preparation

Preoperative preparation for the day of surgery includes appropriate use and timing of personal medications; showering with soap or chlorhexidine the day prior to surgery; absence of makeup, lotion, deodorant, or other skin products; and removal of all jewelry and piercings.

4.2.2 Intraoperative Optimization

The patient is positioned to optimize exposure of the area(s) of the body that will undergo surgery. The monitoring equipment should be positioned to avoid the operative field. The patient should be secured to the operating table to avoid inadvertent movement, which may lead to contamination and iatrogenic injury.

4.2.3 Prophylactic Antibiotics

Antibiotics should be administered less than 2 hours prior to surgery (often the recommendation is within 1 hour) and should not wait until after the incision has been made. This principle was experimented with and proven by Massachusetts General Hospital (MGH) surgeon John Burke. Broad spectrum antibiotics against skin flora (typically gram-positive organisms) or other flora native to a bodily cavity that will be entered (i.e., bowel, genitourinary). The chosen antibiotics should take into consideration the patient's allergies and any adverse responses to prior antibiotic use.

References

1. Berríos-Torres SI, Umscheid CA, Bratzler DW, Leas B, Stone EC, Kelz RR, Reinke CE, Morgan S, Solomkin JS, Mazuski JE, Dellinger EP, Itani KMF, Berbari EF, Segreti J, Parvizi J, Blanchard J, Allen G, Kluytmans JAJW, Donlan R, Schecter WP. Healthcare Infection Control Practices Advisory Committee. Centers for Disease Control and Prevention guideline

for the prevention of surgical site infection, 2017. JAMA Surg. 2017;152(8):784–91. https://doi.org/10.1001/jamasurg.2017.0904. Erratum in: JAMA Surg. 2017;152(8):803. PMID: 28467526.
2. Tanner J, Dumville JC, Norman G, Fortnam M. Surgical hand antisepsis to reduce surgical site infection. Cochrane Database Syst Rev. 2016;2016(1):CD004288. https://doi.org/10.1002/14651858.CD004288.pub3. PMID: 26799160; PMCID: PMC8647968.
3. Global guidelines for the prevention of surgical site infection. Geneva: World Health Organization; 2016. PMID: 27929621.
4. Webster J, Osborne S. Preoperative bathing or showering with skin antiseptics to prevent surgical site infection. Cochrane Database Syst Rev. 2015;2:CD004985. https://doi.org/10.1002/14651858.CD004985.pub5. PMID: 25927093.

Part III
Preparation in the Operating Room-After Anesthesia

Chapter 5
Patient Preparation

David Straughan, Polly-Ann Downey, Michael Yaremchuk, and Dylan Perry

5.1 The Airway

After intubation and before moving the operating room (OR) table and positioning the patient, the patient's airway must be secured.

5.2 Tracheal Tube Security and Access

The senior author's preference is suture or wire stabilization of the endo- or nasotracheal tube to the patient's anatomy. Suture fixation allows intraoperative patient repositioning or head turning without the fear of tube displacement.

D. Straughan
Division of Plastic Surgery, Massachusetts General Hospital, Boston, MA, USA

P.-A. Downey
The Boston Center for Ambulatory Surgery, Inc., Boston, MA, USA

M. Yaremchuk (✉)
Division of Plastic Surgery, Massachusetts General Hospital, and The Boston Center for Ambulatory Surgery, Inc., Boston, MA, USA
e-mail: dr.y@dryaremchuk.com

D. Perry
Harvard Plastic Surgery Residency Program, Boston, MA, USA

© The Author(s), under exclusive license to Springer Nature Switzerland AG 2023
M. Yaremchuk et al. (eds.), *Expertise in the Operating Room*,
https://doi.org/10.1007/978-3-031-30835-2_5

5.2.1 Endotracheal Tube Security

The endotracheal tube is immobilized with wire fixation to the teeth (see Fig. 5.1). A #30 or #32 gauge wire encompassed two adjacent teeth. The ends of the wire were twisted at the outermost edge of the teeth. That positioning allowed the resultant angle at the base of the wire twist to be 90°, which provided less strain on the metal. Twisting wires over the central area of the teeth causes 180° angulation, which results in more strain when twisting and possible wire fracture. Note that in Fig. 5.1, the wire ends are twisted to create a leash of significant length so that the tube is free of the lips.

5.2.2 Nasotracheal Tube Security

For nasotracheal intubation, the tube is sutured to the nasal septum. The septal soft tissues are protected from suture compromise with folded xeroform strips (Fig. 5.2).

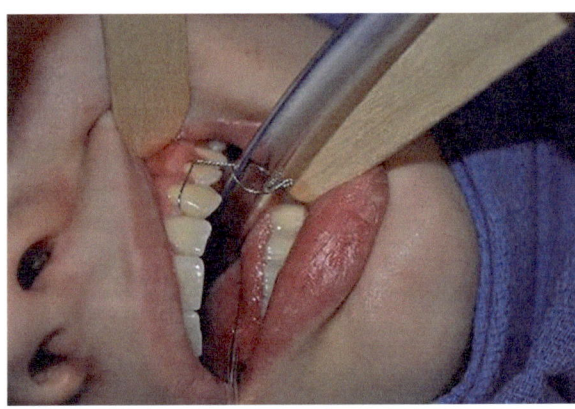

Fig. 5.1 Wire immobilization of the endotracheal tube

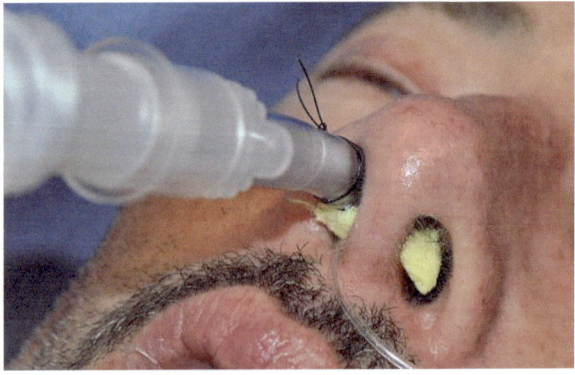

Fig. 5.2 Nasotracheal tube immobilization

Fig. 5.3 The endotracheal tube and ventilator tubing are protected with plastic draping

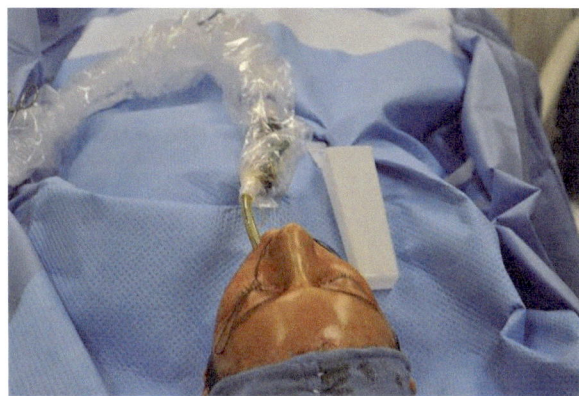

5.2.3 Tracheal Tube Access and Visualization

During patient draping, the endo- or nasotracheal tube and anesthesia tubing are placed in a plastic bag (Fig. 5.3). This combination rests on the drapes, which allows this tubing to be repositioned during the operation. If the distal end of the tracheal tube is disconnected from the connection to the ventilator, it can easily be reconnected intraoperatively without removing the drapes.

Intraoral and intranasal surgery requires the protection of the airway. After nasotracheal or endotracheal intubation, a throat pack is placed to occlude tracheal access from the blood or fluid. The entire intraoperative team must be aware of its presence. It must remain during intraoral suctioning and be removed just prior to extubation.

5.3 Eye Protection

The patient's eye should be protected during any surgery. Lubrication, as shown in Fig. 5.4, prevents corneal desiccation. Taping the lids closed (Fig. 5.5) avoids intraoperative iatrogenic trauma. The status of the eyes and eyelids should always be in the field of the operative surgical or anesthetic teams. Facial operations should include the orbits in the operative field. Procedures not involving the face should be draped to provide facial access to the anesthetic team.

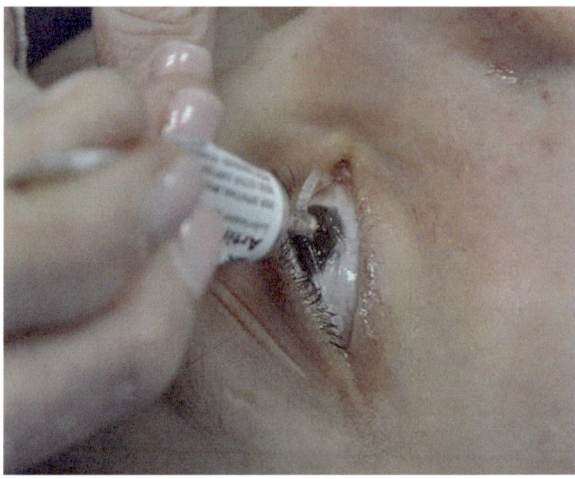

Fig. 5.4 Lubrication covers the cornea from desiccation

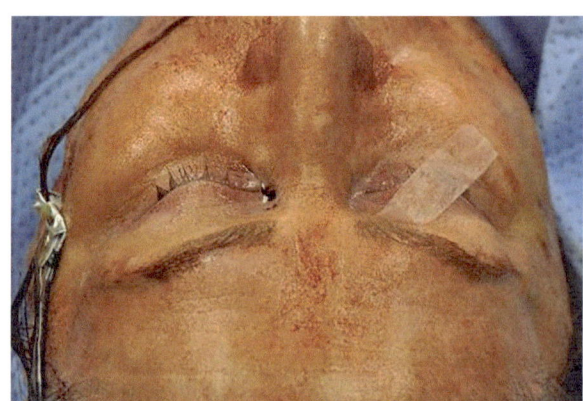

Fig. 5.5 Taping the lower lids closed prevents iatrogenic eye injury

5.4 Ear Canal

Procedures that include the ears in the operative field are subject to preparatory fluids or intraoperative bleeding to seep into the ear canal. Postoperatively, such materials compromise hearing, are uncomfortable, and can be difficult to remove. Placing xeroform or similar strips to occlude the canal eliminates that problem (see Fig. 5.6). After removal of the protection within the ear canal and before the end of the procedure, the ear canal can be suctioned carefully to assure ear canal patency.

Fig. 5.6 A xeroform strip is being placed to occlude the ear canal from access to perioperative fluids

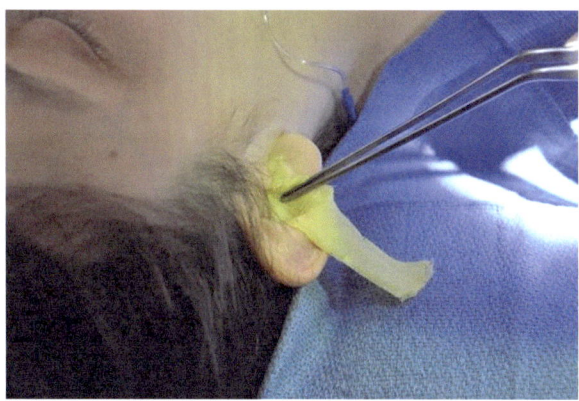

5.5 Patient Positioning

Once the patient is anesthetized and stable, the OR table is positioned in a place that provides optimal access to the surgical team. It assures direct access to overhead lighting, the ventilator, and instrumentation.

Patient positioning is coordinated between the surgeon, anesthesiologist, and circulating nurse. The patient is positioned to optimize access to the operative site. Positioning in the prone or lateral position is more time-consuming during positioning but assures optimal site and optimal operative technique.

Compromised exposure and positioning predicts compromised surgery.

Immobilized soft tissues between skeletal prominences and underlying support structures (operating bed, arm boards, and additional supporting tables) compromise circulation, which may lead to pressure necrosis with tissue loss. Not only are the soft tissues at risk, but also motor and sensory nerves are at risk. These pressure sores can be avoided by cushioning the areas of concern with gel padding (Fig. 5.7). Table 5.1 presents positions, surgical sites, and pressure points to be protected.

Patient positioning should also avoid traction injury to the extremities. Once positioned, the torso and extremities must be secured to avoid intraoperative displacement, which may be hidden by drapes.

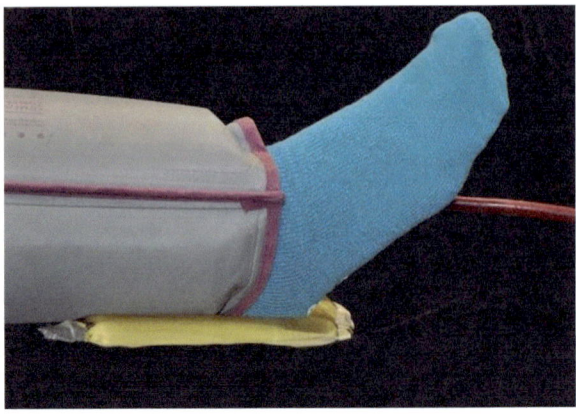

Fig. 5.7 Heel is protected from pressure necrosis with an underlying gel pad. (Note: Venodyne boots have been placed)

Table 5.1 Commonly utilized patient positioning in the operating room

Position	Surgical sites	Pressure points to be protected
Supine	Head, neck, thorax, abdomen, extremities occiput, scapula, sacrum, heels	Ulnar nerve, heels, occiput, sacrum
Prone	Spine, buttocks/anus	Face, breasts, genitalia, knees, toes
Lateral	Thorax ear, acromion, iliac crest, greater trochanter, knee, ankle	
Lithotomy	Anus, perineum, genitals, inner thigh	Occiput, scapula, sacrum, heels, ulnar nerve, perineal nerve

Adapted from Medtronic Patient Positioning Manual

5.6 Skin Preparation

Skin preparation reduces the number of bacterial colonies on the skin.

5.6.1 Debridement

The first step is to remove any gross debris, skin slough, eschar, or drainage attached to sutures or keratoses by scrubbing the area. Scrubbing should be performed gently to avoid skin breaches. Hair thought to compromise surgical exposure should be removed with clippers (not with a razor) or preoperatively with a depilatory agent. The removal of debris and hair should be performed before the surgeon or assistant scrubs in.

5.6.2 Solutions

According to the Food and Drug Administration (FDA), an ideal skin prep agent should substantially reduce transient microorganisms; possess a broad spectrum of antimicrobial properties; be fast acting; have persistent, cumulative activity; and be nonirritating to the skin. Current skin preparation products include povidone-iodine (Betadine), combined alcohol and chlorhexidine solutions (ChloraPrep), iodine povacrylex with isopropyl alcohol (DuraPrep), and para-chloro-meta-xylenol (PCMX). These agents are also typically used for the surgeon and assistant's hand preparation. Centers for Disease Control and Prevention (CDC) guidelines support the use of alcohol-based prep solutions (combined with another antiseptic, such as chlorhexidine) over iodine solutions due to their broad spectrum, fast onset, and long-lasting effect [1–3]. A randomized control trial in the New England Journal of Medicine (NEJM) found lower rates of infection with chlorhexidine-alcohol than povidone-iodine in clean-contaminated surgery [3]. Alcohol-based prep should not be used in open wounds and mucous membranes due to the risk of tissue damage to normal tissue and mucous membranes (Table 5.2).

After debridement, the skin should then be dried with a towel before applying the skin site preparation. Principles of applying the solution to avoid contamination include the following:

1. Prepare a wide surgical field. For breast surgery, the entire chest from the navel to the neck and the bilateral lateral chest down to the operating table should be included and free of any contaminated objects. The limb is usually prepared circumferentially for surgery.
2. Prepare in order starting from clean areas and moving to dirty areas. Infected or contaminated areas should be prepped after clean areas if possible.
3. Prepare from central to lateral. First, prepare the area of focus, then extend out radially to prepare the borders of the surgical field.
4. Allow iodine solutions to dry to obtain maximal efficacy. Alcohol solutions that are pooled or not fully dried risk fire when exposed to electrocautery.

Table 5.2 Activity and considerations for preoperative patient skin antiseptics

	Aqueous iodine/iodophors (10%) [1]	Chlorhexidine gluconate (CHG) (4%) [4]	[a]Alcohol (70–91.3%) [5]	Alcoholic iodine/iodophors [5]	CHG-alcohol [5]
Mechanism of action [1–5]	Oxidation/substitution with free iodine	Disrupts cell membrane	Denatures cell wall proteins; concentration determines effectiveness	See aqueous iodine/iodophors and alcohol	See CHG and alcohol
Effectiveness against microorganisms [1–5]	Gram + and gram − bacteria, tubercle bacillus, fungi, and viruses	Gram + and gram − bacteria, yeasts, and some viruses	Gram + and gram − bacteria, mycobacteria, fungi, and viruses	See aqueous iodine/iodophors and alcohol	See CHG and alcohol
Rapidity of action [1–5]	Moderate	Moderate	Most rapid	Rapid	Rapid
Residual activity [1–5]	Moderate	Excellent	None	Moderate	Excellent
Use on eyes, ears, or mouth [1, 4, 6]	Yes, ears and mouth; for the eyes, use 5% ophthalmic solution	No, eyes and ears; can cause corneal damage or deafness if contacts the middle ear; for the mouth, use 0.12% CHG oral rinse	Yes, ears No, eyes and mouth; can cause corneal damage or nerve damage	No; can cause corneal damage or nerve damage	No; can cause corneal damage; can cause deafness if contacts the middle ear
Use in the genital area [1, 4, 6]	Yes, use with caution in patients susceptible to iodism [7]	No [6]	No	No	No
Use internally [1, 4, 6]	No, external use only	No, external use only; do not use on wounds that involve more than superficial layers of skin	No, external use only	No, external use only; do not use on open wounds	No, external use only; do not use on open wounds

(continued)

Table 5.2 (continued)

	Aqueous iodine/iodophors (10%) [1]	Chlorhexidine gluconate (CHG) (4%) [4]	[a]Alcohol (70–91.3%) [5]	Alcoholic iodine/iodophors [5]	CHG-alcohol [5]
Contradictions [1, 4, 6]	Sensitivity or allergy to drug or any ingredients	Sensitivity or allergy to drug or any ingredients; do not use for lumbar puncture or in contact with meninges	Sensitivity or allergy to drug or any ingredients	Sensitivity or allergy to drug or any ingredients	Sensitivity or allergy to drug or any ingredients; do not use for lumbar puncture or in contact with meninges
Cautions [1, 4, 6]	Use with caution in patients susceptible to iodism (e.g., patients with thyroid disorders, neonates, pregnant women, lactating mothers); prolonged exposure may cause irritation; inactivated by blood	Use with caution in premature infants or in infants younger than 2 months old, may cause chemical burns	Flammable	Flammable. Do not use in infants younger than 2 months old. Use with caution in nursing mothers. Use caution when removing adhesive drapes to avoid skin inquiry	Flammable; use with caution in premature infants or in infants younger than 2 months old; may cause a chemical burn

[a] Isopropyl alcohol (70–91.3%) is classified as Category I for the preparation of the skin prior to an injection
(References [1–8])

5.7 Draping

The surgical site is draped after it has been prepped and dried. The field should include adequate adjacent visibility. This perspective avoids possible damage to adjacent structures (e.g., the eye). It can also provide adequate access to contralateral structures for assessment of symmetry.

The surgical field is first isolated with sterile (often blue or green) towels. The folded blue towel should be placed onto the surgical field, then slide toward the nonsterile area. When the blue towels are placed in their desired position, they can be secured using adhesive drapes, staples, or towel clips. Depending on the location of the surgical site, the surgeon may further secure blue towels by placing a few staples onto the patient to prevent the risk of contamination due to the necessary movement of the surgical site during the operation. An adhesive clear plastic dressing (e.g. "thousand drape") is an effective way to immobilize the blue towel, preventing operative field contamination if the towel is dislodged (Fig. 5.8).

5.7.1 Drapes

Sterile drapes come in a variety of shapes to optimize visualization and maintain the sterility of different anatomical locations. To avoid drape contamination, two surgical team members should drape the patient.

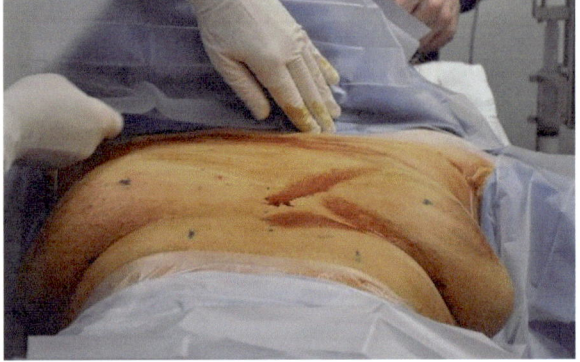

Fig. 5.8 The transparent towel has an adhesive on one edge. The adhesive contacts both the skin and the blue towel edge. This immobilizes the towel's position and prevents the exposure of an unsterile area in the operative field

5.8 Tubes and Cords

After the sterile field is established, suction tubing, cords for electrocautery, and/or drills should be placed next, should be identifiable, and should not be kinked. Tubing and cords should be connected to their outlets by the circulator so that they are functioning at the beginning of the operation.

5.9 Monopolar Electrocautery: The Bovie and the Grounding Pad

An electrosurgical unit (ESU) is a generator capable of creating alternating current at a high frequency to induce heat energy capable of achieving coagulation by drying out cells or to cut tissues by the vaporization of cells.

Monopolar electrocautery is usually referred to as "the Bovie," in respect of its inventor, William T. Bovie. The Bovie's generator sends electrical current to a desired area of the body for treatment. The current travels through the patient back to a grounding pad before it reaches the generator to create the circuit (Fig. 5.9).

The grounding pad is responsible for the safe return of current to the electrosurgical generator and provides a path of low resistance and low current (Fig. 5.10).

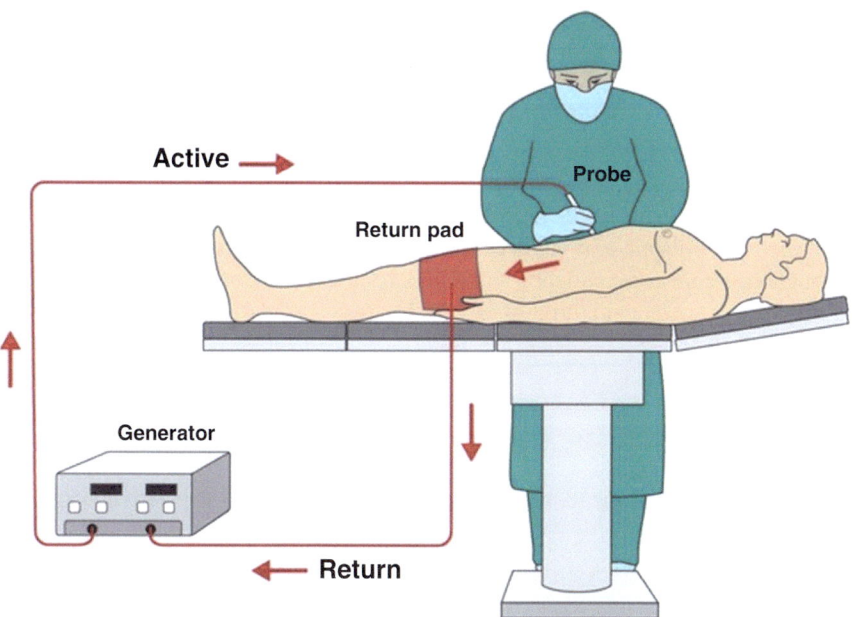

Fig. 5.9 Diagram of the Bovie shows electric current from the generator traveling through the patient back to the grounding pad before it reaches the generator to complete the circuit

Fig. 5.10 Grounding pad attached to the upper thigh of a patient

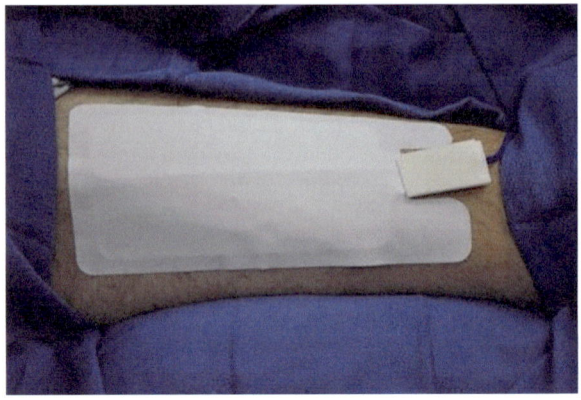

The risk of burn is increased when the contact quality between the patient and the grounding pad is poor.

This can occur if the grounding pad is placed against an unshaven area, an area covered with moisturizers, a bony prominence, scar tissue, or an area with little soft-tissue mass. For that reason, contact area grounding pads should be positioned over dry, shaven, and well-vascularized tissue surfaces.

If the grounding pad is improperly positioned or dislodged, piercings could act as a return pathway for the ESU and cause burns.

5.10 Intermittent Pneumatic Compression (IPC) Devices (Venodyne Boots) (Fig. 5.7)

Intermittent pneumatic compression (IPC) devices are used to help prevent blood clots in the deep veins of the legs during surgery. The devices use cuffs around the legs that fill with air and squeeze the patient's legs. This increases blood flow through the veins in the patient's legs and helps prevent blood clots. IPC is one way to help prevent deep vein thrombosis (DVT).

References

1. Zamora JL. Chemical and microbiologic characteristics and toxicity of povidone-iodine solutions. Am J Surg. 1986;151(3):400–6.
2. Berríos-Torres SI, Umscheid CA, Bratzler DW, Leas B, Stone EC, Kelz RR, Reinke CE, Morgan S, Solomkin JS, Mazuski JE, Dellinger EP, Itani KMF, Berbari EF, Segreti J, Parvizi J, Blanchard J, Allen G, Kluytmans JAJW, Donlan R, Schecter WP. Healthcare Infection Control Practices Advisory Committee. Centers for Disease Control and Prevention guideline for the prevention of surgical site infection, 2017. JAMA Surg. 2017;152(8):784–91. https://

doi.org/10.1001/jamasurg.2017.0904. Erratum in: JAMA Surg. 2017;152(8):803. PMID: 28467526.
3. Darouiche RO, Wall MJ Jr, Itani KM, Otterson MF, Webb AL, Carrick MM, Miller HJ, Awad SS, Crosby CT, Mosier MC, Alsharif A, Berger DH. Chlorhexidine-alcohol versus povidone-iodine for surgical-site antisepsis. N Engl J Med. 2010;362(1):18–26. https://doi.org/10.1056/NEJMoa0810988. PMID: 20054046.
4. Lim K-S, Kam PCA. Chlorhexidine—pharmacology and clinical applications. Anaesth Intensive Care. 2008;36(4):212–21.
5. Reichman DE, Greenberg JA. Reducing surgical site infections: a review. Rev Obstet Gynecol. 2009;2(4):212–21.
6. DailyMed US National Library of Medicine. http://dailymed.nim.nih.gov/. Accessed 14 Jul 2014.
7. American College of Obstetrics and Gynecologists Women's Health Care Physicians, Committee on Gynecologic Practice. Committee Opinion No. 571: Solutions for surgical preparation of the vagina. Obstet Gynecol. 2013;122(3):718–20.
8. US Food and Drug Administration. Tentative final monograph for healthcare antiseptic drug products proposed rule. Fed Regist. 1994;59(116):31402–52.

Part IV
Surgery

Chapter 6
Logistics and Ergonomics

David Straughan, Imran Ratanshi, Julianna Paniss, and Michael Yaremchuk

6.1 Equipment

6.1.1 Operating Table

The position of the operating table provides operative access for the entire operative team. The surgeon's visibility is paramount but equally includes that of the anesthetist, scrub nurse, and circulating staff. To be effective, each member of the team should be attuned to each part of the operation. The operating team resembles that of a winning baseball team where every team player responds appropriately to each pitch and the batter's response.

The patient and operative field must be positioned, prepared, and draped appropriately [1]. The operative field should include adequate adjacent field visibility. This perspective avoids possible damage to adjacent structures (e.g., the eye).

D. Straughan · I. Ratanshi
Division of Plastic Surgery, Massachusetts General Hospital, Boston, MA, USA

J. Paniss
The Boston Center for Ambulatory Surgery, Boston, MA, USA

M. Yaremchuk (✉)
Division of Plastic Surgery, Massachusetts General Hospital, and The Boston Center for Ambulatory Surgery, Inc., Boston, MA, USA
e-mail: dr.y@dryaremchuk.com

© The Author(s), under exclusive license to Springer Nature Switzerland AG 2023
M. Yaremchuk et al. (eds.), *Expertise in the Operating Room*,
https://doi.org/10.1007/978-3-031-30835-2_6

6.1.2 Lighting

Effective lighting requires proper positioning of the overhead ceiling lamps [2]. Today's operating rooms are equipped with a major overhead light and additional mobile arms with elbows, which allow precise positioning. The operating room table is positioned to best utilize the lighting system. The major lamp is positioned directly above the operative field so that the center of attention is visible to the entire team. A secondary light is placed behind the operating shoulder of the surgeon to parallel their sight line (Fig. 6.1).

Today's overhead operating room light fixtures are generally light-emitting diodes (LED). LED lights are long-lasting, white-light producing, with good shadow control that do not produce excessive heat.

6.1.3 Team Positioning

The surgeon must be positioned to comfortably access the operative field and overhead lighting and utilize his assistants. The surgical assistant and scrub nurse or scrub technologist positioning should allow their visualization of the field and assistance to the surgeon without inhibiting the surgeon's performance. This positioning will be mandated by the nuances of the surgical procedure. The scrub nurse or scrub technologist and the table with the commonly used instruments must be close enough to effectively hand an instrument.

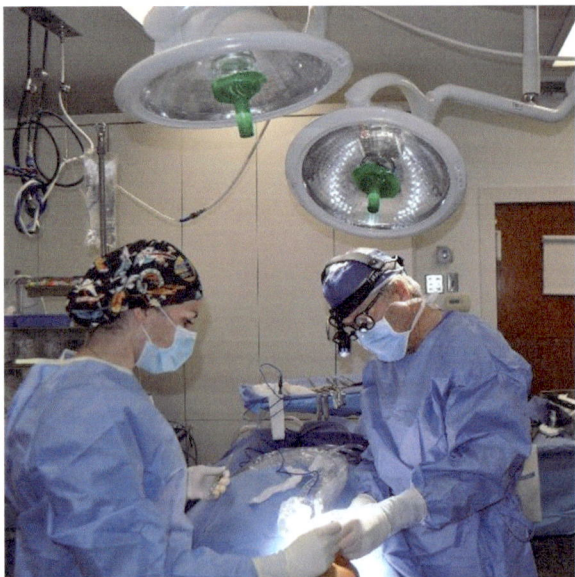

Fig. 6.1 Overhead lighting arrangement with a major lamp positioned directly above the operative field and a secondary lamp behind the right shoulder of the surgeon to parallel his sight line

6.1.4 Operative Assistance

An operation has one surgeon who designs and orchestrates the procedure. An assistant surgeon optimizes the surgeon's operative maneuvers and does not engage in a secondary endeavor unless requested by the primary surgeon.

The operative personnel assist and take cues from the surgeon. This includes providing appropriate instrumentation and operative field exposure with tissue retraction and hemostasis. A professional operative team knows the goal and sequence of the operation, thereby minimizing repetition and optimizing efficiency [3, 4].

6.1.5 Retraction

The surgeon's visibility of the operative field requires the retraction of adjacent tissues or structures [5]. The positioning of retractors, although requested and positioned by the surgeon, is maintained by the other members of the surgical team. Retractors are designed in many shapes and sizes appropriate for a given situation. The professional scrub nurse or scrub technician after viewing the operative situation will provide the appropriate size and length of a requested type of retractor's blade length or width or its handle length.

The retractor blade length that is appropriate to the depth of the wound should be chosen.

A blade length that protrudes beyond the wound edges technically adds to the depth of the wound, thereby hindering surgical access. On the other hand, a blade length inadequate to reach the depth of the wound will limit surgical exposure (Fig. 6.2).

Once the retractor is positioned by the surgeon, it is the assistant's job to maintain the instrument in a static or dynamic position. To do so, the assistant must be observing the operative field, along with the surgeon's motions. A delicate, crucial maneuver by the surgeon may require the operative field to be still. On the other

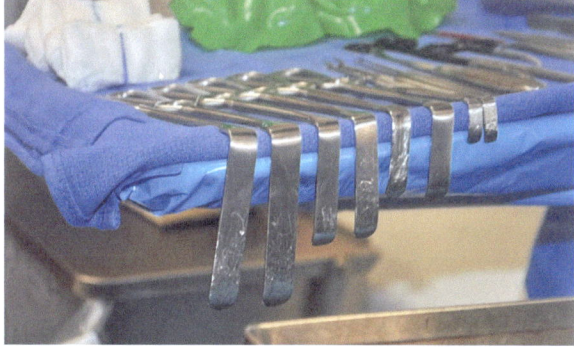

Fig. 6.2 Note that the instruments' design has various blade lengths appropriate for the depths of wounds

hand, when the surgeon is enlarging the scope of the operative field, ongoing active retraction aids the surgeon by continuously adding visibility during the surgeon's dissecting process.

Traction by the surgeon and countertraction by the assistant improve field exposure by better exposing tissue planes.

6.2 Instrument Selection and Passing

The efficiency of an operation will be influenced by the instruments available for a given procedure. The surgical technologist must have all instruments on the Mayo stand organized and available for use. This implies their knowledge of the goal of the operation and its sequence. In addition, it is important to follow the surgeon's actions to anticipate needs and requests.

The Mayo stand should be positioned so that the technologist can easily access instruments and also can easily observe the surgeon's actions.

The surgeon should not have to look away from the field to accept instruments.

Instruments are placed to the surgeon:

- Firmly into the surgeon's hands
- Ready to be used
- If curved, curved in the direction of intended use
- If ringed, with the box locked
- In such a way that the curved surgical needle is positioned with the needle about 1/8 inch from the tip of the needle holder and with the needle one third from the swage (Fig. 6.3)

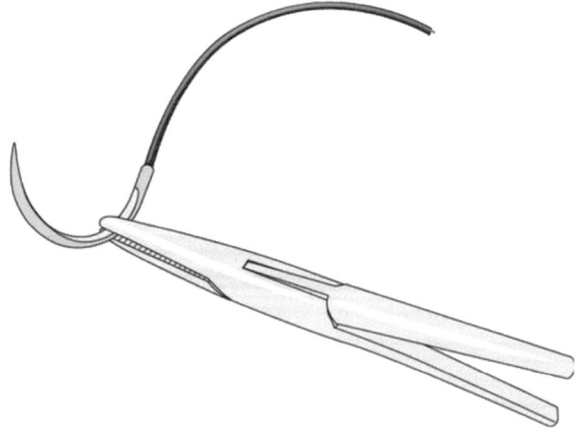

Fig. 6.3 The curved surgical needle is positioned with the needle about 1/8 inch from the tip of the needle holder and with the needle one third from the swage

Instruments should be passed in a functional position to the surgeon. In addition, the size and design of the instrument should be chosen by the scrub nurse or scrub technologist and should be appropriate for the instrument's use. This implies that the scrub nurse or scrub technologist is in synchrony with the procedure.

6.3 Hemostasis (Suctioning)

A fundamental role of the assistant is suctioning blood that otherwise obscures the surgeon's visibility of the operative field.

> *Suctioning does not limit or stop blood loss. The effective assistant suctions blood at the interface of the surgeon's instrument and the involved tissue.*

Suctioning in an area away from the operative field is not productive and can be distracting.

6.4 The Operation's End

6.4.1 The Patient

Before dressing the wound, the operative site should be cleansed of any blood *or* preparation fluid on the patient, particularly along the wound suture closure. Blood oozing through the closure becomes part of the wound suture line. Subsequent suture removal adjacent to these wound closure imperfections disrupts the wound closure, causing interruptions with prolonged healing and aesthetic disharmony. The initial response to their surgery is often impacted by the obvious professional attention of their surgical dressing, hospital setting, and hospital attire.

6.4.2 The Instruments

Before drapes are removed, all instruments, sharps, and cords are returned to the back table or Mayo stand to avoid instrument loss and to assure a complete instrument count. All sharps should be placed in the designated sharp container and discarded in the sharps' bin. Until the dressing is placed, instruments should remain sterile and available. When the operation is finished, the scrub nurse or scrub technologist and the circulator should make a final closing count.

Soiled surgical instruments should not be soaked in normal saline on the back table to avoid corrosion due to the effect of chloride on stainless steel. The soiled instruments should be separated from nonsoiled instruments and sprayed with an enzymatic solution to start the breakdown process of bioburden.

References

1. Medtronic. Patient positioning. Available https://www.essote.fi/wp-content/uploads/sites/2/2016/10/patient-positioning-medtronic-copy-yhteensopivuustila.pdf. Accessed 27 December 2020.
2. Elias-Fogle L. Why is operating room light important? Available https://www.steris.com/healthcare/knowledge-center/surgical-equipment/operating-room-lighting#:~:text=%20Types%20of%20Light%20Bulbs%20%201%20Halogen,LED%20bulbs%20offer%20much%20longer%20life%2C...%20More%20. Accessed 27 December 2020.
3. Epstein S, Sparer EH, Tran BN, Ruan QZ, Dennerlein JT, Singhal D, Lee BT. Prevalence of work-related musculoskeletal disorders among surgeons and interventionalists: a systematic review and meta-analysis. JAMA Surg. 2018;153(2):e174947. https://doi.org/10.1001/jamasurg.2017.4947. Epub 2018 Feb 21. PMID: 29282463; PMCID: PMC5838584.
4. Steele PR, Curran JF, Mountain RE. Current and future practices in surgical retraction. Surgeon. 2013;11(6):330–7. https://doi.org/10.1016/j.surge.2013.06.004. Epub 2013 Aug 6. PMID: 23932799.
5. Hall S, Quick J, Hall AW. The perfect surgical assistant: calm, confident, competent and courageous. J Perioper Pract. 2016;26(9):201–4. https://doi.org/10.1177/175045891602600903. PMID: 29328813.

Chapter 7
Fire

David Mattos, Michael T. Bailin, and Michael Yaremchuk

Up to 90% are caused by electrocautery and overall, OR fires comprise 1.9% of the surgical malpractice cases since 1985 [1].

7.1 The "Fire Triad"

An operating room (OR) fire requires three components, known as the "fire triad" or the "fire triangle." The triad includes (1) an oxidizer, (2) an ignition source, and (3) a fuel source (Fig. 7.1).

7.1.1 Oxidizer

An oxidizer provides a fire-friendly environment. In the OR, oxygen and nitrous oxide function as oxidizers. Oxidizer-enriched environments within the OR exist within the airway-ventilator circuit and in areas where open oxygen sources (e.g., nasal cannula, mask) are concentrated by the configuration of the surgical drapes.

D. Mattos
Harvard Mass General Brigham Plastic Surgery Residency Program, Boston, MA, USA

M. T. Bailin
The Boston Center for Ambulatory Surgery, Boston, MA, USA

M. Yaremchuk (✉)
Division of Plastic Surgery, Massachusetts General Hospital, and The Boston Center for Ambulatory Surgery, Inc., Boston, MA, USA
e-mail: dr.y@dryaremchuk.com

Fig. 7.1 An illustration of the fire triad depicts the three fundamental requirements: (1) an oxidizer, (2) an ignition source, and (3) a fuel source

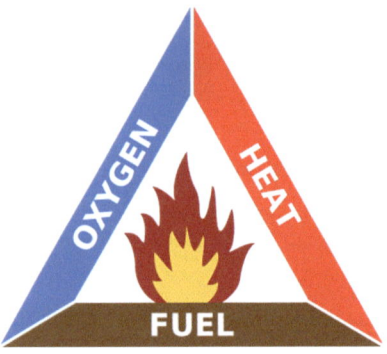

Any increase in oxygen concentration above room air, as well as any presence of nitrous oxide, is considered oxidizer enriched.

7.1.2 Heat or Ignition Source

An ignition source provides the energy to start a fire. Whether it is a mechanical, electrical, or heat source, each has the ability to start a fire in the right environment. Heat or ignition sources include electrocautery, drills and burrs, lighting instruments, electrical pads, electrical wires, lasers, and probes.

7.1.3 Fuel

Fuel includes anything that can burn. In the OR, the list of fuel includes alcohol-containing prep solutions, sponges, drapes, dressings, tubing, gowns, packaging materials, gastrointestinal tract gasses, hair, blankets, endoscopic instruments, and gloves.

7.2 Fire Prevention

Fire prevention requires every member of the operative team to be aware of the factors in the environment that can lead to a fire and its avoidance. The sparking and heating associated with a monopolar electrical surgical unit, commonly referred to as the Bovie, can provide ignition to cause a fire in the operating room environment.

Oxidizers such as oxygen and nitrous oxide provide a fire-friendly OR environment. They exist within the airway-ventilator circuit and in areas where open oxygen can increase in oxygen concentration above room air. Surgical fields enhanced with oxygen markedly facilitate flammability. A standard blue towel used as a surgical drape will ignite 16 times faster (0.1 s versus 1.6 s) in an environment of 100% oxygen [2].

Supplemental oxygen (the oxidizer) is rarely required yet regularly overutilized in conscious sedation cases.

Open oxygen delivery, via a mask or nasal cannula, is often unnecessarily applied for superficial surgical procedures on the shoulders, neck, face, and head, precisely where the drapes will concentrate excess and dangerous oxygen gas. Adding an oxidizer to complete the fire triad is a choice that should rarely be made. For patients who absolutely require supplemental oxygen (e.g., patients on home oxygen), a strong argument exists to use an airway device that will ensure no leakage of oxygen into the atmosphere (e.g., laryngeal mask or supraglottic airway).

There are many fuel sources that can burn in the OR, including alcohol-containing prep solutions, sponges, drapes, towels, dressings, tubing, gowns, packaging materials, gastrointestinal tract gasses, skin, hair, blankets, endoscopic instruments, and gloves.

Daane and Toth listed these strategies to minimize the risk of an OR fire [3].

7.2.1 Oxidizer

- Use protected endotracheal tubes when operating in the vicinity.
- Use only air or air/oxygen mixtures in anesthetic gasses.
- Do not use nitrous oxide, particularly if performing bowel surgery.
- Do not tent the surgical drapes in a way that would allow oxygen to build.
- Use an incise drape with adhesive for procedures above the clavicle to keep combustible gasses below the drapes.
- Suction out the gasses from the mouth of an intubated patient in oropharyngeal surgery.

7.2.2 Heat or Ignition Source

- Place the cautery in its holster when not in use. The same holds true for all other devices that can be an ignition source.
- Do not use cautery settings that lead to sparks.
- Never use a cautery to enter the trachea.
- Avoid supplemental oxygen for at least 1 min before cautery use on the face or neck.
- Use nonconductive plastic clamps to clamp holsters to the surgical drapes.

- Turn off light sources when not in use.
- Do not allow fiber optic cables to come in contact with drapes or other flammable materials.

7.2.3 Fuel

- Use water-soluble (not oil-based) solutions or gels to cover hair.
- If using alcohol-based skin preparations, allow it to dry completely before placing surgical drapes or towels (wait for 3 min minimum).
- Use fire-resistant surgical drapes.
- **Wet all sponges used in oropharyngeal surgery.**

7.3 Specific Guidelines for Using a LASER [4]

1. Avoid using supplemental oxygen for face procedures by using nerve blocks with intravenous sedation.
2. Limit density and pulse duration as much as possible.
3. Use the standby mode when not in use.
4. If there is no metal laser-safe endotracheal tube, wrap the tube with wet gauze or aluminum foil.
5. Place moist towels around the treatment area to avoid igniting surrounding materials.
6. Use metal corneal shields to prevent corneal thermal injury.

7.4 Responding to an OR Fire

A useful figure for the sequence of dealing with an operating room fire has been produced by the American Society of Anesthesiologists [5]. The OR team should always be on the lookout for early signs of OR fires, which include smoke, heat, patient movement under drapes, discoloration of drapes or breathing tubes, flash, unusual sounds, and unusual odors. After identifying that there is a fire present, the procedure must be immediately stopped, and the management phase begins (different for airway fires and nonairway fires).

Airway fires require the immediate removal of the endotracheal tube, stopping of the flow of oxygen and other gasses, and removal of sponges or other flammable materials from the airway. After doing so, saline should be poured into the airway. After the fire is stopped, one can reestablish ventilation and the airway but should avoid oxidizer-enriched atmospheres, if at all possible. After securing the airway, the removed endotracheal tube should be inspected for fragments, which could suggest a retained object inside the airway. Bronchoscopy should also be considered.

Nonairway fires first require the stopping of all gasses and the removal of all burning or flammable materials. Saline should be poured over burning materials as a first attempt to extinguish the fire.

When the fire is out, make sure to maintain ventilation of the patient and assess for possible inhalation injury signs, which include facial burns, blistering or swelling of the oropharynx, hoarseness, stridor, mucosal lesions of the upper airway, and carbonaceous sputum.

The entire OR staff should be advised immediately of any fire. If small, the fire should be stopped immediately with a gloved hand or saline. If the fire cannot be stopped after the first attempt, the OR's CO_2 fire extinguisher, which all staff should be facile with, should be used to attempt to extinguish the fire. If the fire spreads to other parts of the room, the patient should be evacuated, the OR door closed, and the gas supply stopped.

All OR staff should be periodically trained and drilled in fire awareness, prevention, and treatment. A useful OR poster is provided by the American Society of Anesthesiologists, which describes appropriate operating room fire response in an easy-to-follow diagram [5]. Necessary fire response equipment and supplies include saline, CO_2 fire extinguisher, additional endotracheal tubes and masks, rigid laryngoscope, replacement airway breathing circuit and lines, and replacement drapes. These should be readily available during all surgeries.

7.4.1 OR Fire Resources

Additional useful resources with checklists, posters, and videos can be found on the website of the Association of periOperative Registered Nurses (AORN) [6]. An emergency response manual that can be used for OR fires and other similar emergencies is also provided free of charge by Stanford University.

References

1. Brooks M. Surgical fire prevention. 2018. Available https://www.medscape.org/viewarticle/898018.
2. Culp WC Jr, Kimbrough BA, Luna S. Flammability of surgical drapes and materials in varying concentrations of oxygen. Anesthesiology. 2013;119(4):770–6. https://doi.org/10.1097/ALN.0b013e3182a35303. PMID: 23872933.
3. Daane SP, Toth BA. Fire in the operating room: principles and prevention. Plast Reconstr Surg. 2005;115(5):73e–5e. https://doi.org/10.1097/01.prs.0000157015.82342.21. PMID: 15809576.
4. Rohrich RJ, Gyimesi IM, Clark P, Burns AJ. CO2 laser safety considerations in facial skin resurfacing. Plast Reconstr Surg. 1997;100(5):1285–90. https://doi.org/10.1097/00006534-199710000-00034. PMID: 9326794.

5. American Society of Anesthesiologists. A report by the American Society of Anesthesiologists Task Force on operating room fires; practice advisory for the prevention and management of operating room fires. Anesthesiology. 2008;108:786–801; quiz 971-2. https://doi.org/10.1097/01.anes.0000299343.87119.a9.
6. Fire Safety: Association of Perioperative Registered Nurses. 2020. Available https://www.aorn.org/guidelines/clinical-resources/tool-kits/non-member-tool-kits/fire-safety-tool-kit-nonmembers.

Part V
The Surgeon's Tools

Chapter 8
Surgeon's Instruments

Eric J. Wenzinger, Timothy J. Irwin, and Michael Yaremchuk

Instruments are classified by their function.

8.1 Cutting and Dissecting

Sharp-edged instruments are designed to cut, dissect, separate, or excise tissue.

8.2 Scalpel: Surgical Blades and Handles

8.2.1 Surgical Blades

Historically, surgical scalpels were single-piece knives. Repeated use and heat sterilization blunted their use, requiring frequent intraoperative sharpening. Surgical scalpels consisting of a handle and a detachable blade were invented by Morgan Parker in 1915. C. R. Bard was the medical supplier who first manufactured this

---

Supplementary Information The online version contains supplementary material available at https://doi.org/10.1007/978-3-031-30835-2_8.

E. J. Wenzinger · T. J. Irwin
Harvard Mass General Brigham Plastic Surgery Residency Program, Boston, MA, USA

M. Yaremchuk (✉)
Division of Plastic Surgery, Massachusetts General Hospital, and The Boston Center for Ambulatory Surgery, Inc., Boston, MA, USA
e-mail: dr.y@dryaremchuk.com

© The Author(s), under exclusive license to Springer Nature Switzerland AG 2023
M. Yaremchuk et al. (eds.), *Expertise in the Operating Room*,
https://doi.org/10.1007/978-3-031-30835-2_8

instrument, hence the still common use of the "Bard-Parker" scalpel. The detachable blade was made for easy exchange of a sharp and inexpensive cutting edge. Scalpel blades have evolved from chromium and nickel-coated carbon steel blades to high-carbon stainless steel, which provide high corrosion resistance with the preserved ability to hone and maintain a razor-sharp edge [1].

8.2.1.1 Standard Blades

Blade shapes and sizes are numbered from #9 to #36. The blades that are commonly used in clinical practice and illustrated in Fig. 8.1 include the 10, 15, 15c, 11, 20, and Beaver blades.

#10 Blade: The #10 blade, with its curved cutting edge, is used for large skin incisions.

#15 Blade: The #15 blade is significantly smaller in size and is useful for short shallow incisions.

#15c Blade: This #15c blade variant is designed for small, radius curvature incisions frequently used in periodontal applications.

#11 Blade: The #11 blade is an elongated triangular blade sharpened along the hypotenuse edge with a strong, pointed tip ideal for initial skin puncture or tiny deep incisions.

#22 Blade: The #22 blade is a larger version of the #10 blade with a curved cutting edge and a flat, sharpened back edge. It is used for large skin incisions in both cardiac and thoracic surgery.

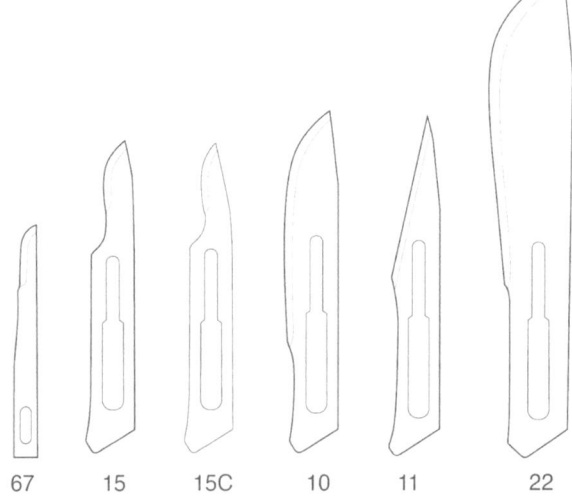

Fig. 8.1 Commonly used surgical blades and their respective sizes. Most instrument sets include #3 and #7 knife handles

Beaver blades: These blades are secured by a small diameter round handle. This delicate design is facile for working in concavities and with small delicate areas such as the eyelids and hands.

8.2.2 Knife Handles

Knife handles are designed in various lengths and widths to accommodate the type of blade and the surgical field. The handles are designed and numbered to secure certain scalpel blades. For example, #3 or #7 handles fit blades with the numeric prefix "1" (e.g., #10, #11, #12, #15), while #4 handles fit larger blades with the numeric prefix "2" (e.g., #20, #21, #22, #23, #24).

Knife handle images are shown in the following figures. See Figs. 8.2, 8.3, and 8.4.

#7 Handles are longer, ergonomically shaped handles appropriate for work in deep cavities. See Fig. 8.4.

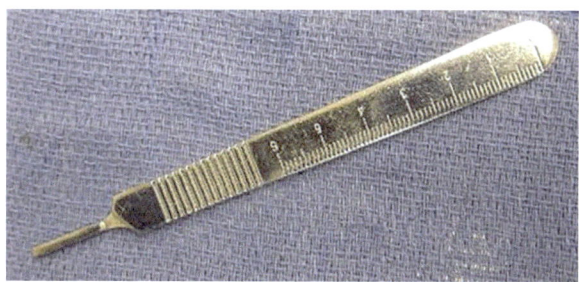

Fig. 8.2 #3 Handle

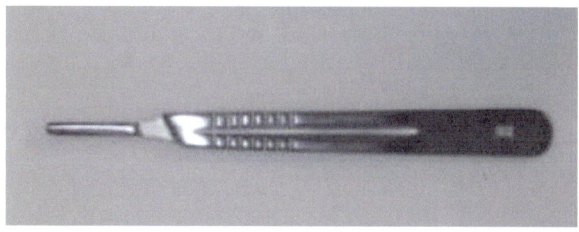

Fig. 8.3 #4 Handle

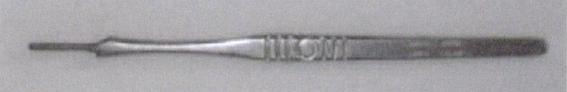

Fig. 8.4 #7 Handle: a long, ergonomically shaped handle that is appropriate for work in cavities

Fig. 8.5 Beaver handle

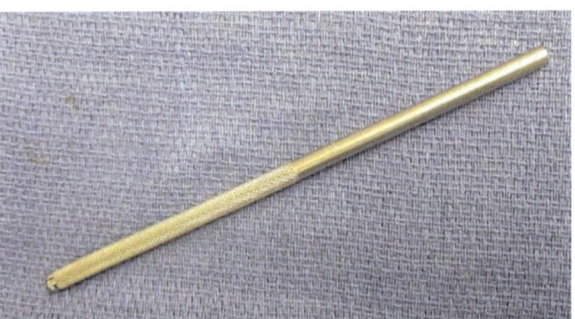

Beaver handles are solely used for beaver microsurgical blades and consist of round handles ranging from 2" to 6" in length. They typically have a textured grip and a collet distally to secure the disposable blades (see Fig. 8.5). The Beaver blade is shown in Fig. 8.5.

8.3 Scissors

Scissors are hand-operated shearing tools. A pair of scissors consists of a pair of metal blades pivoted so that the sharpened edges slide against each other when the handles opposite to the pivot are closed. The blades of scissors may be straight, angled, or curved with tips either pointed or blunt. Handles may be long or short. Scissors are used for cutting or dissecting various soft tissues. Their size, shape, and caliber are designed to address their specific usage and should be used for their intended purpose. The term "scissor" is the singular version of the same noun. It is almost never used, the same way that bellows are nearly always referred to in the plural. As noted above, the default singular form would be a pair of scissors. Below are the most frequently used scissors (Figs. 8.6, 8.7, and 8.8).

8.3.1 Mayo Scissors

The Mayo brothers, William Mayo (1861–1939) and Charles Mayo (1865–1939), were general surgeons who, with their father, William W. Mayo, founded the Mayo Clinic. The Mayo family was given credit for inventing these scissors. These heavy scissors can be straight or curved and are designed for dissecting thicker or more fibrous tissue.

Fig. 8.6 A pair of straight Mayo scissors

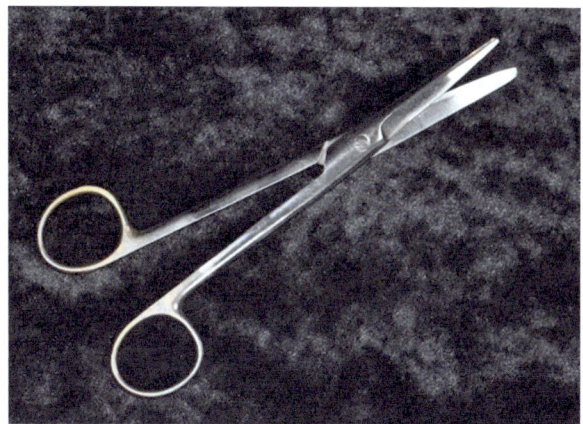

Fig. 8.7 Metzenbaum scissors. Note that the handle-to-blade length is much longer than that of Mayo scissors

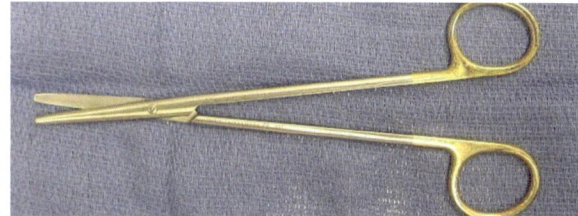

Fig. 8.8 Straight iris scissors

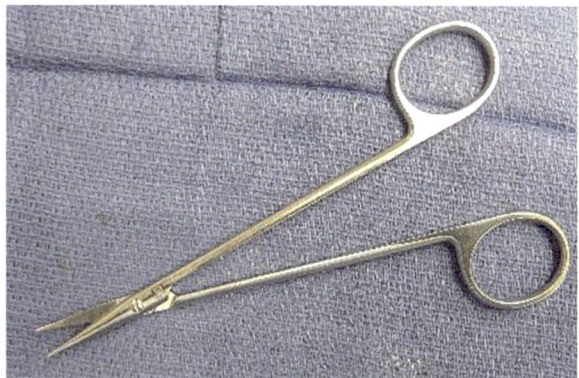

8.3.2 Metzenbaum ("Metz") Scissors

Myron Metzenbaum (1876–1944) was an otolaryngologist who practiced in Cleveland. He was known to have small hands (size 6 gloves) and designed a pair of scissors with smaller handles. Initially designed for tonsillectomy, their clinical application has extended far beyond the field of otolaryngology for the use of tissue more delicate than that intended for Mayo scissors. In addition to a lesser scale, the

Metzenbaum scissor handle to blade length is much longer than that of Mayo scissors. There are many variations of scissors with this basic design with a longer handle-to-blade ratio and are therefore labeled Metzenbaum scissors (see Fig. 8.7).

8.3.3 Small, Delicate Scissors

Smaller, delicate scissors are very sharp and fine tipped with minor specific variations. They include both curved and straight varieties. Among others, smaller, delicate scissors include Iris, Stevens tenotomy, and Potts' scissors.

8.3.3.1 Iris Scissors

Iris scissors were initially intended for ophthalmologic use but are used more widely for fine dissection and incisions.

8.3.3.2 Tenotomy Scissors

Similar to iris scissors, tenotomy scissors are sharp, fine-tipped scissors for cutting and dissecting delicate tissue, such as blood vessels, nerves, and tendons. They are larger than iris scissors, ranging anywhere from 4″ to 8″ in length. Stevens tenotomy scissors have a traditional single-hinge mechanism. The Westcott tenotomy scissors have a dual leaf spring and hinge mechanism. Pott tenotomy scissors are larger with longer handles ranging from 6″ to 8″ in length.

8.4 Forceps

Forceps and clamps are designed to grasp and hold a tissue in place without injuring surrounding tissues. Forceps have two basic designs. Tissue forceps stabilize tissues but require the continuous grasp and maintenance of the surgeon. Locking forceps are termed clamps. Their mechanism allows the stable purchase of tissue or vessel without pressure applied by the surgeon.

8.4.1 Toothed vs. Smooth

The distribution of force applied when using toothed and nontoothed forceps is quite different, as is their ultimate effect on the tissue they directly contact. There is a greater amount of force applied at the distal teeth as they are the first point of contact, resulting in more of a pincer grip as opposed to a crushing grip of nontoothed forceps where the force is more equally distributed between the tines. For this reason, nontoothed smooth forceps should not be used routinely when handling skin to avoid crushing the skin edges and causing tissue necrosis. Similarly, toothed forceps are not typically used when handling blood vessels or other delicate subcutaneous tissue since they may tear or puncture the vessel wall.

8.4.1.1 Toothed Forceps

8.4.1.1.1 Adson

Alfred W. Adson (1887–1951) was a neurosurgeon and innovator, who pioneered the surgical sympathectomy for the treatment of hypertension. He introduced Adson forceps, which remain widely used for fine dissections across surgical specialties. Adson forceps are characterized by a single interlocking set of teeth (Fig. 8.9a). They are used for fine dissecting and for relatively atraumatic tissue handling, particularly skin. Nontoothed variants (smooth Adsons) were produced later by instrument companies unaware of the surgical history (Fig. 8.9b).

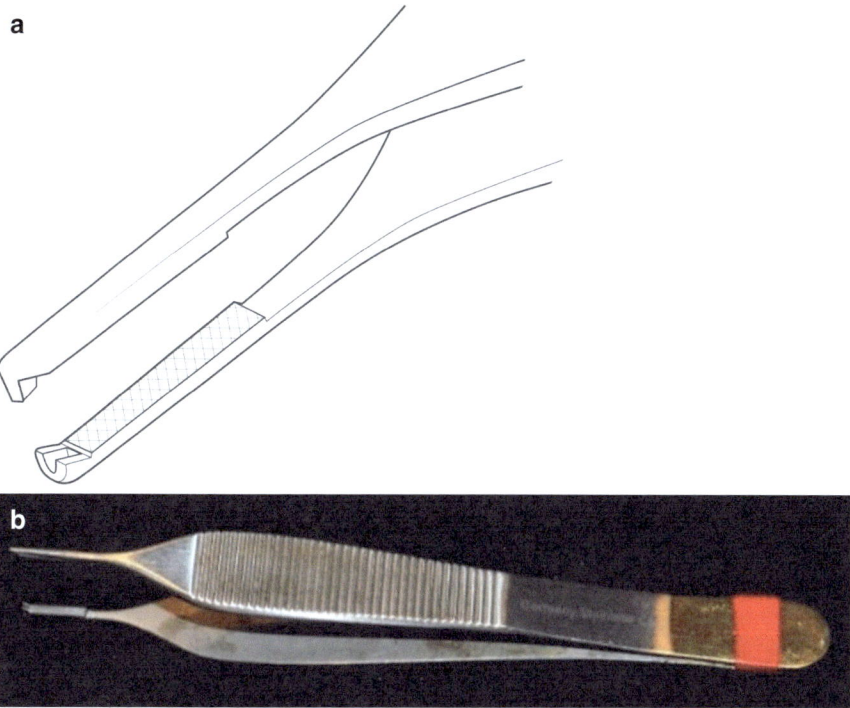

Fig. 8.9 (**a**) Illustration of the locking tip design of the Adson forceps. (**b**) Clinical example of Adson smooth forceps

8.4.1.1.2 Adson-Brown

Rather than teeth, these forceps have multiple interdigitating ridges along their distal aspect (see Fig. 8.10). This design not only provides an additional grip but is also more traumatic when handling tissues. For that reason, many surgeons avoid their use during skin closure.

8.4.1.1.3 Bishop-Harmon ("Iris")

These forceps are very similar to Adson forceps but are more delicate in scale and are exceptionally fine tipped. They have flat handles, which typically have three holes in them (see Fig. 8.11).

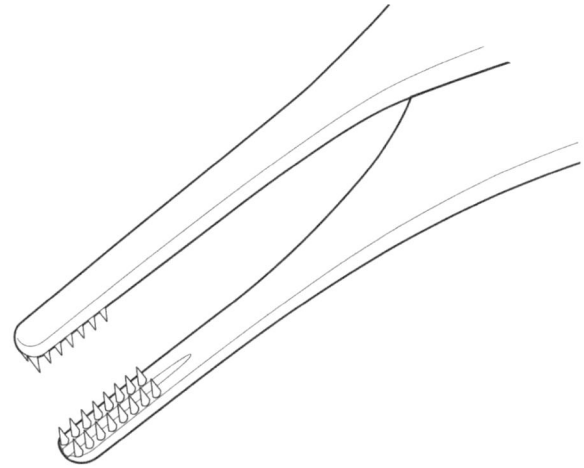

Fig. 8.10 Tip design of Adson-Brown forceps

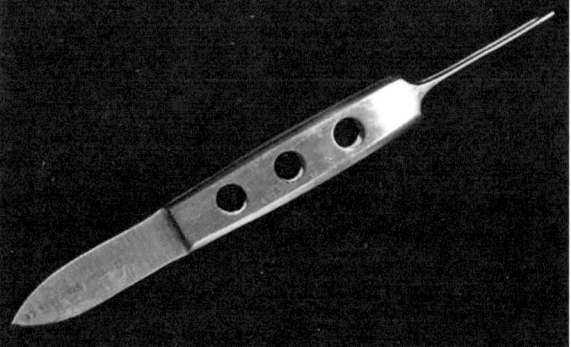

Fig. 8.11 Iris forceps are fine toothed and typically have three holes in the handle

Fig. 8.12 Tip design of Bonney forceps

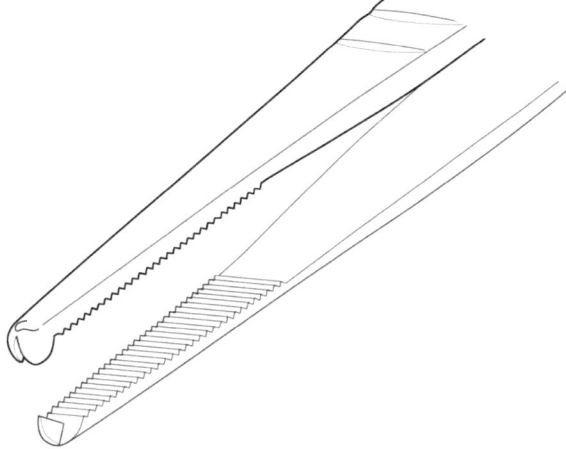

Fig. 8.13 Tip design of rat tooth forceps

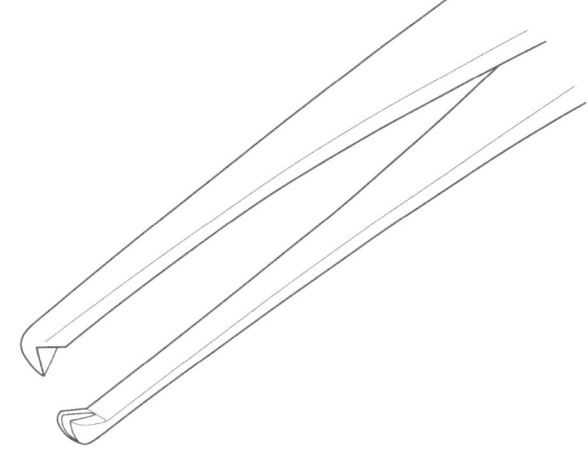

8.4.1.1.4 Bonney

Victor Bonney (1872–1953) was a British gynecological surgeon who designed these forceps particularly for handling round ligaments. These forceps are heavier-toothed forceps with additional transverse ridges along the distal tines (see Fig. 8.12). Their design and scale are ideal for purchasing fascia and dense connective tissue.

8.4.1.1.5 Rat Tooth

Rat tooth forceps are larger forceps with a single set of interdigitating teeth, named according to their likeliness to rodent teeth (see Fig. 8.13). These forceps are used for grasping thick/tough tissue such as fascia and dense breast tissue.

8.4.1.2 Smooth Forceps

8.4.1.2.1 DeBakey

Michael DeBakey (1908–2008) was a cardiac and vascular surgeon responsible for several contributions. His contributions include polyethylene terephthalate (Dacron) vascular grafts, Mobile Army Surgical Hospitals (MASHs) during World War II, the first successful carotid endarterectomy, and DeBakey forceps.

DeBakey forceps are nontoothed and are characterized by a more coarsely, ridged grip segment distally, which can be oriented transversely or parallel to the forceps axis (see Fig. 8.14). In general, they come in larger sizes than most forceps. This design minimizes trauma to vessel walls and is used routinely for vascular procedures.

8.4.1.2.2 Nonvascular

Forceps that are smooth without ridges are often used to position intraoperative devices (see Fig. 8.15). They are ideal for use during suture removal since they provide relatively broad opposing surfaces or sutures, which provide a secure purchase of the suture end.

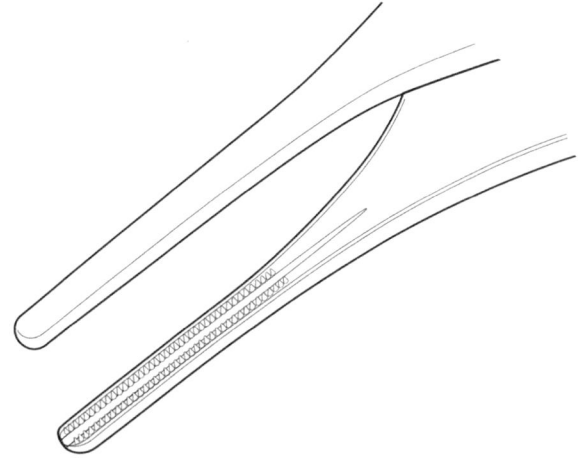

Fig. 8.14 Tip design of DeBakey forceps

Fig. 8.15 Tip design of smooth forceps

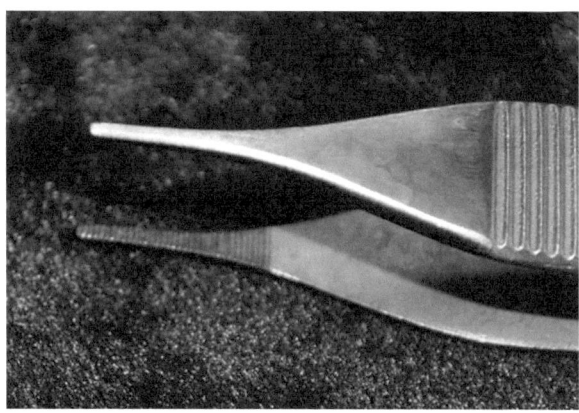

8.5 Clamps (Locking Forceps)

8.5.1 Clamps That Secure Tissue

8.5.1.1 Allis

Oscar Huntington Allis (1836–1921), a general surgeon in Philadelphia, designed these forceps to use during primary bowel anastomosis. With prescience, he wrote: "I do not care to recommend these instruments simply as aids in intestinal work…," knowing their potential application would extend beyond intra-abdominal surgery. These forceps are characterized by their straight arms with curved jaws, which meet along a parallel mildly toothed surface distally (see Fig. 8.16).

8.5.1.2 Babcock

William Babcock (1872–1963), a general surgeon in Philadelphia, introduced these forceps for intra-abdominal operations. His surgical innovation extended beyond abdominal surgery, introducing novel techniques for treating varicose veins and the "soup bone" cranioplasty. These forceps are characterized by their looped jaws and do not have teeth or transverse ridges for grasping, making them less traumatic than Allis forceps. Their looped jaws are curved toward each other and meet along a smooth, round surface distally (see Fig. 8.17). These were initially designed for grasping bowel but are used more broadly in clinical practice.

8.5.2 Clamps That Crush Tissue

These clamps are characterized by transverse ridges along their jaws (see Fig. 8.18). Clamps come in different sizes and configurations, depending on their clinical application.

8.5.2.1 Jacobson ("Mosquito")

These small straight or curved forceps are of fine caliber (see Fig. 8.19). They are often used to secure small vessels prior to their ligature or electrocoagulation.

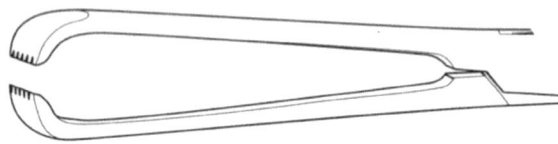

Fig. 8.16 Tip design of Allis forceps

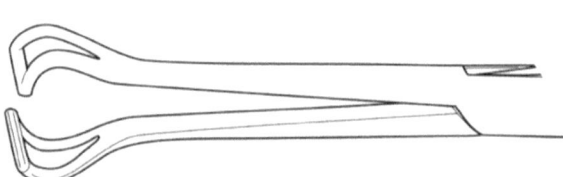

Fig. 8.17 Tip design of Babcock forceps

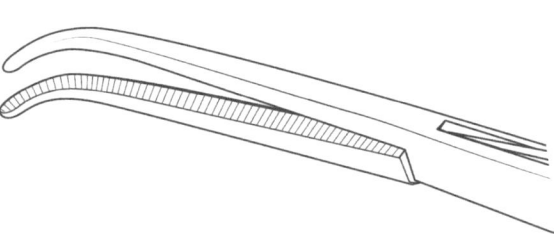

Fig. 8.18 The characteristic transverse ridges of the various clamps designed to crush tissues. The tip design of a Schnidt clamp is illustrated

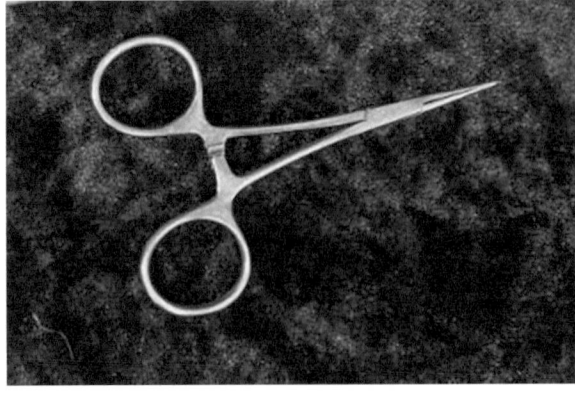

Fig. 8.19 Jacobson or "mosquito" forceps

8.5.2.2 Crile ("Snap")

George Washington Crile (1864–1943) was a general surgeon and founding member of the American College of Surgeons (ACS). He designed a small hemostatic clamp utilized during neck dissections. The Crile, or "Snap," forceps are straight or curved fine-tipped forceps with transverse ridges along their entire length. They are larger than Jacobson forceps and are similarly used to provide hemostasis for small to medium vessels.

8.5.2.3 Kelly

Howard Kelly (1858–1943) was the first professor of gynecological and obstetrical surgery at the Johns Hopkins Hospital. He used locking forceps to control larger blood vessels and diffusely oozing tissues during uterine surgery. The Kelly forceps may be straight or curved.

8.5.2.4 Kocher

Emil Kocher (1841–1917) was a general surgeon and researcher who invented this hemostatic clamp. He was known for his popularization of the aseptic surgical technique and was awarded the Nobel Prize in 1909 for his contributions to the field of thyroid surgery. Available with straight or curved jaws, Kochers are characterized by large teeth distally and transverse ridges along the entire length of their jaws (see Fig. 8.20). They are used for grasping and retracting fascia or dense connective tissue.

8.5.2.5 Mixter ("Right Angle")

Both Samuel Mixter (1855–1919) and William Mixter (1809–1884) were neurosurgeons at the Massachusetts General Hospital (MGH). The distal aspect of the Mixter, or "Right Angle," jaws are curved at angles ranging between 45° and 90°, allowing dissection or hemostasis in difficult-to-reach sites. These forceps vary in size from fine to broad tips. Like Jacobson and Crile forceps, they have transverse ridges along the entire length of their jaws.

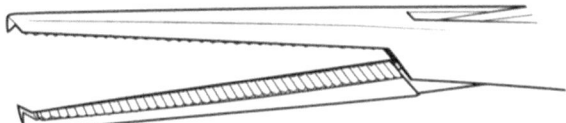

Fig. 8.20 The Kocher design has large teeth distally and transverse ridges along the entire length of their jaws

8.5.2.6 Tonsil "Schnidt"

The Tonsil, or "Schnidt," clamps have long handles with curved jaws that have transverse ridges along their entire length (see Fig. 8.21). They were initially intended to apply packing in the tonsillar fossae following tonsil removal but are used more widely in clinical practice.

8.6 Exposing and Retracting

8.6.1 Simple Retractors

Retractors maintain tissues in desired positions to provide exposure to the operative site. Shapes, sizes, as well as blade and handle lengths vary according to clinical necessity. Deep cavities require longer retractors. Short retractors are intended for relatively superficial exposure depths. Retractors may be handheld or self-retaining.

8.6.2 Handheld Retractors

8.6.2.1 Army-Navy

These retractors have a central grip with a blade on each end. The blades are often of different lengths (Fig. 8.22).

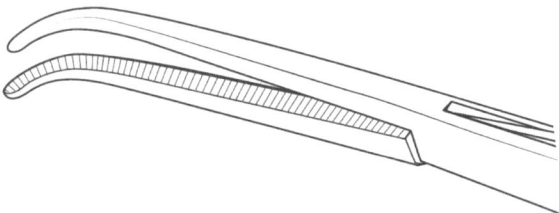

Fig. 8.21 Tip design of Schnidt clamp

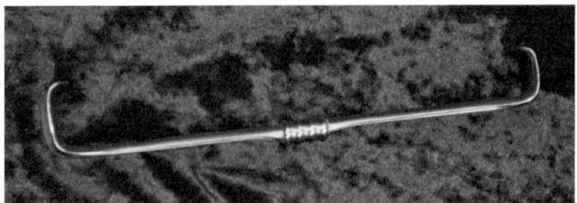

Fig. 8.22 An army-navy retractor

8.6.2.2 Senn-Miller ("Senn")

Nicholas Senn (1844–1908) was a general surgeon based in Chicago who was known for his contributions to pancreatic and plastic surgery. The Senn-Miller, or "Senn," retractor has two different types of blades on a central grip (see Fig. 8.23). On one side is a finger-like flat-bladed retractor that is bent at 90° with a short-curved lip distally. The opposite side has a rake with three tines, which can be blunt or sharp. *The curved ends of each side are directed 180° opposite of each other, unlike Army-Navy retractors.*

8.6.2.3 Hooks

These are sharp, hook-shaped retractors with one or two tines used to retract skin edges (see Fig. 8.24). Their length (varying according to the operative field) allows the assistant to retract without obstructing the surgeon's field of view.

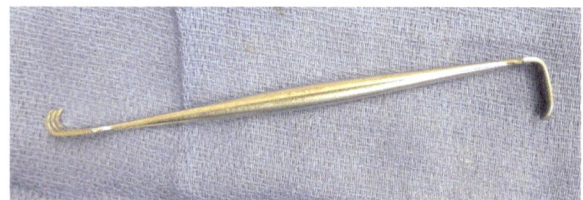

Fig. 8.23 A Senn retractor

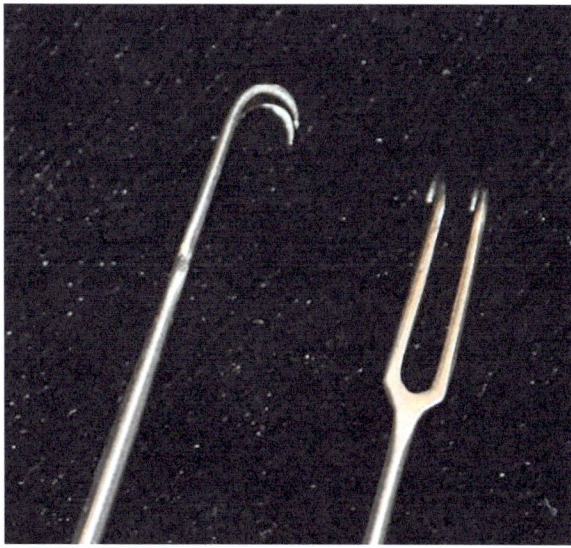

Fig. 8.24 Example of a double hook retractor

8.6.2.4 Richardson ("Abdominal Wall") Retractor

Maurice Richardson (1851–1912) was a general surgeon and former chief of surgery at the MGH. It was designed to retract the abdominal wall when working on the bowel or visceral structures. The handles can be looped or round and typically have ergonomic indentations for the assistant's fingers. The blade length ranges between 1 and 2 inches.

8.6.2.5 Deaver

These retractors have long, flat-curved blades intended to hold large tissue flaps. They are shaped like a question mark with blade sizes ranging from 1 to 3 inches in width and up to 13 inches in length (see Fig. 8.25). They can have round ergonomically shaped handles or flat handles with a curve at the end intended to prevent the assistant's finger or thumb from sliding up the instrument.

8.6.3 Self-Retaining Retractors

8.6.3.1 Weitlaner

Franz Weitlaner (1872–1944) was an Austrian surgeon who practiced in the remote village of Ottenthal. He often operated with minimal assistance, hence his design of this self-retaining retractor in 1905. These retractors are useful when a surgeon is operating alone or requires other types of assistance from the surgical assistant. The Weitlaner has long, curved arms that meet distally with curved fork-like tines or flat blades, depending on the clinical field necessary for retraction. Proximally, a ratcheting mechanism keeps the arms in the desired locked position (see Fig. 8.26a, b). A variant with finger-like projections has sides that interdigitate when closed.

8.6.3.2 Gelpi

Maurice Gelpi (1883–1939) was a surgeon who specialized in obstetrics and gynecology at Tulane University. He introduced the Gelpi retractor in 1913 as a perineal retractor. This retractor operates using the same ratcheting mechanism as the

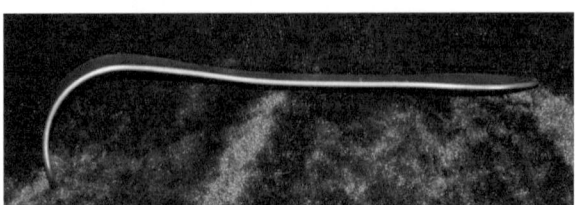

Fig. 8.25 Example of a Dever retractor

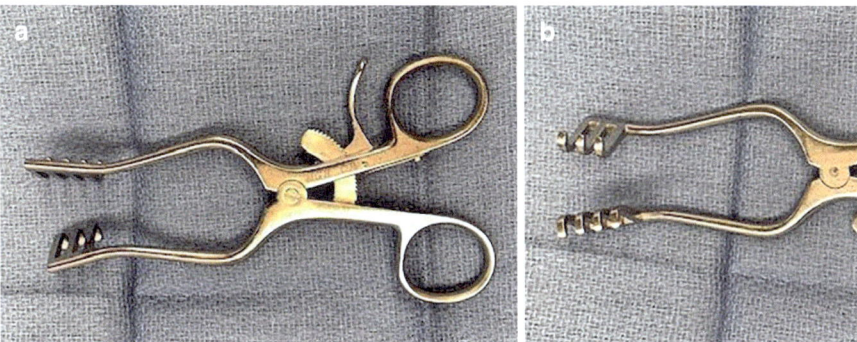

Fig. 8.26 (**a**) Weitlaner retractor top view. (**b**) Weitlaner retractor bottom view

Weitlaner retractor but has single tines at the end of the two long curved arms, which are pointed outward toward the tissue. The shape of the instrument somewhat resembles elephant tusks and is used for small surgical sites with targeted tissue to be retracted.

8.6.3.3 Bookwalter and Lonestar

John Bookwalter (1939–present), a graduate of Harvard Medical School and a general surgeon in Vermont, invented the Bookwalter retracting system, patented in 1979. Alternatively, Medicalis produces a similar product called the Lonestar. Both of these devices are considered retracting systems. Both systems are customizable. The Bookwalther design consists of a central ring composed of stainless steel, while in the Lonestar design, the central ring is plastic. The ring for each of these retracting systems is suspended over the surgical site. The ring of the Bookwalter retractor is secured in a sterile fashion to the bed rail via stainless steel adaptors, including a variety of retracting blades that can be attached to the ring. The Lonestar system does not attach to the bed but is suspended to the surgical site using a series of elastic stay retractors consisting of sharp metal hooks secured within elastic bands. These systems are primarily used for abdominal surgeries.

8.7 Suctioning

8.7.1 Yankauer

Sidney Yankauer (1872–1932), an otolaryngologist based at Mount Sinai Hospital in New York, invented this instrument for suctioning in the mouth. The Yankauer is the most commonly used suction tip in clinical practice. With a long curved neck and a flared rounded tip, it is suited for wide suctioning larger volumes of fluids (see Fig. 8.27).

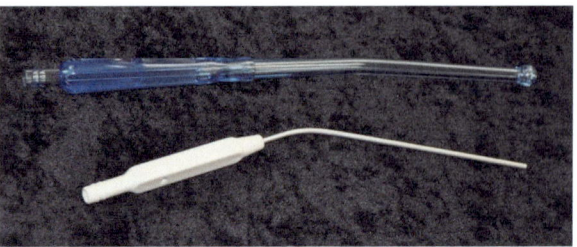

Fig. 8.27 Yankauer suctioning tool above, with Frazier suctioning apparatus below

8.7.2 Pediatric ("Tonsil")

This suction tip is a variation of the Yankauer suction tip design and is typically composed of metal. As the name "Tonsil" implies, it is meant for use in the oropharynx; however, it can be used outside of the mouth in places where a conventional Yankauer would be too bulky.

8.7.3 Frazier

This suction tip is less obtrusive than a traditional Yankauer suction tip and is appropriate for smaller surgical sites. The narrow lumen of the suction tubing is typically the same caliber along its entire length and offers greater resistance to airflow, resulting in less powerful suctioning (see Fig. 8.27). Suction is controlled by a small hole (finger valve) on the handle.

8.8 Needle Holders

Needle holders vary according to the type of needle used, determining their length, scale, and tip design. Webster, Crilewood, and Mayo are the most popular types of needle holders. Webster needle holders are for delicate use and have smooth purchasing surfaces. Sutures greater than 5-0 will damage the tip and purchase of a Webster needle holder. Sutures smaller than 0 size will not be secured by the larger-scale Hegar needle holder (see Fig. 8.28). Hegar needle holders are more robust with textured surfaces to assure a secure grip (see Fig. 8.28).

Fig. 8.28 Purchasing end of a Hegar needle holder

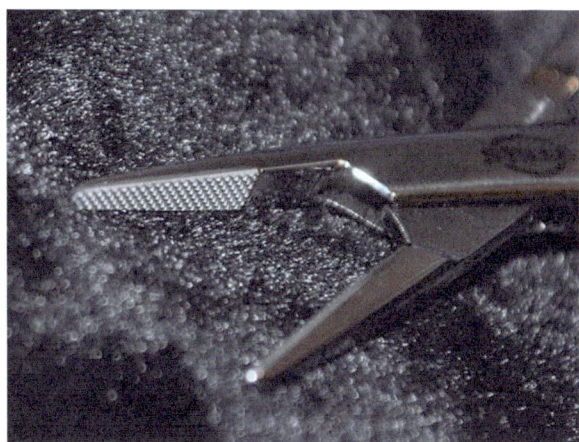

Reference

1. Ailawadi G, Nagji AS, Jones DR. The legends behind cardiothoracic surgical instruments. Ann Thorac Surg. 2010;89:1693–700.

Chapter 9
Sutures and Needles

Brent B. Pickrell and Michael Yaremchuk

9.1 Sutures

Sutures can be classified according to their size and biomechanical properties, tendency to be absorbed, and physical configuration. These attributes determine suture selection for a given surgical indication.

9.2 Suture Diameter

Suture size equates to suture diameter and is denoted using the USP (United States Pharmacopeia) numbering system. This system centers around the "0" suture. Modern sutures range from #5 (heavy-braided sutures for orthopedics) to #11-0 (fine monofilament sutures for ophthalmic surgery). Atraumatic needles are manufactured in all shapes for most sizes. The actual diameter of thread for a given USP. size differs depending on the suture material class (Table 9.1).

Supplementary Information The online version contains supplementary material available at https://doi.org/10.1007/978-3-031-30835-2_9.

B. B. Pickrell
Harvard Mass General Brigham Plastic Surgery Residency Program, Boston, MA, USA

M. Yaremchuk (✉)
Division of Plastic Surgery, Massachusetts General Hospital, and The Boston Center for Ambulatory Surgery, Inc., Boston, MA, USA
e-mail: dr.y@dryaremchuk.com

© The Author(s), under exclusive license to Springer Nature Switzerland AG 2023
M. Yaremchuk et al. (eds.), *Expertise in the Operating Room*, https://doi.org/10.1007/978-3-031-30835-2_9

Table 9.1 Varying sizes of synthetic sutures according to their US Pharmacopeia denotation, metric gauge, diameter (in millimeters), and material class

USP designation	Collagen diameter (mm)	Synthetic absorbable diameter (mm)	Nonabsorbable diameter (mm)	American wire gauge
11-0			0.01	
10-0	0.02	0.02	0.02	
9-0	0.03	0.03	0.03	
8-0	0.05	0.04	0.04	
7-0	0.07	0.05	0.05	
6-0	0.1	0.07	0.07	38–40
5-0	0.15	0.1	0.1	35–38
4-0	0.2	0.15	0.15	32–34
3-0	0.3	0.2	0.2	29–32
2-0	0.35	0.3	0.3	28
0	0.4	0.35	0.35	26–27
1	0.5	0.4	0.4	25–26
2	0.6	0.5	0.5	23–24
3	0.7	0.6	0.6	22
4	0.8	0.6	0.6	21–22
5		0.7	0.7	20–21
6			0.8	19–20
7				18

9.3 Biomechanical Properties

Suture material will determine its biomechanical properties.

9.3.1 Tensile Strength

Tensile strength is determined by suture diameter. As defined by the United States Pharmacopeia (USP), tensile strength is the necessary weight to break a suture divided by the cross-sectional area of the suture. The surgeon should select the suture of the smallest caliber that will accomplish adequate tissue coaptation. In general, for a given suture size, sutures of synthetic materials are stronger than those of natural materials.

9.3.2 Memory

Memory refers to the inherent capacity of a material to return to its original shape after being manipulated. Sutures with high memory ratings are typically stiffer, more difficult to handle, and more susceptible to becoming untied than sutures with less memory. Most monofilament synthetic sutures exhibit a high degree of memory compared to their multifilament counterparts. Sutures of materials with high memory require more knots to prevent untying.

9.3.3 Elasticity

Elasticity refers to a suture's intrinsic ability to return to its original length after being stretched. Sufficient elasticity allows the suture to expand to accommodate wound edema without leading to strangulation (ischemia) or tissue injury. Similarly, elasticity allows the suture to recoil during wound contraction or maintain wound edge apposition once edema has subsided. Elasticity is not to be confused with *plasticity*, which refers to a material's ability to retain its new length and shape following manipulation. As opposed to a suture material with high elasticity, one with high plasticity will not return to its initial length after the deforming force has been removed. As such, after tissue swelling has subsided, a suture with significant plasticity may be too loose to keep wound edges opposed.

9.3.4 Coefficient of Friction

The coefficient of friction describes how easily the suture will pass through tissue, both during placement and if/when the suture is removed. Sutures with low frictional values, such as poliglecaprone 25 or polypropylene, slide through tissue easily and, for that reason, are commonly selected for running subcuticular or percutaneous closures. The lower is the coefficient of friction for a given suture, the more likely it is that a resultant knot may slip and unravel. As a result, these materials require more throws to enhance knot strength and security. Braided sutures have higher coefficient of friction values than monofilament sutures.

9.3.5 Knot Security

Knot security refers to the ability of suture material to remain tied. When a knotted suture becomes untied, the consequences can be catastrophic; as such, *knot security* is paramount. Knot security can be affected by suture type, knot configuration, suture memory, and the number of throws. *Knot strength* is calculated by determining the force necessary to cause a knot to slip. This is directly proportional to the suture's coefficient of friction, number of throws, and ability to stretch. Choosing a suture with a high coefficient of friction and introducing additional throws to increase the contact surface area within the knot both increase the amount of friction that must be overcome to permit slippage. Similarly, placing square throws, which increase knot friction, results in greater knot strength and decreases the risk of wound dehiscence.

9.3.6 Tissue Reactivity

The amount of foreign body inflammation evoked by a suture material within a wound defines its tissue reactivity. All suture materials elicit some element of foreign-body response, regardless of their chemical composition. Natural materials (e.g., silk or plain gut) incite a more robust inflammatory response than synthetic materials (e.g., polypropylene or polyglactin 910). The amount of suture material implanted determines the tissue reaction. Because the foreign-body inflammatory reaction of suture materials adversely affects wound healing, the surgeon must balance the advantages and disadvantages of each suture material with regard to their size, composition, and absorption profile.

9.4 Mono- and Multifilament Sutures

Strand composition is a consideration in suture characteristics.

9.4.1 Monofilament

Configuration with a single strand lessens the surface area, thereby inciting less tissue reaction. A monofilament suture is more resistant to bacterial adhesion, making it more appropriate for use in a contaminated field. Because it is less reactive and glides through tissues more easily, skin and intradermal closures are appropriate for its use. The disadvantages of monofilament sutures include increased memory, more difficult handling, and inferior knot security. As a result, more throws are needed with monofilament materials to create a secure knot. Examples of common monofilament sutures include polydioxanone (PDS II (Ethicon, Inc.)), poliglecaprone 25 (Monocryl, Ethicon, Inc.), nylon (Ethilon, Ethicon, Inc.), and polypropylene (Prolene, Ethicon, Inc.).

9.4.2 Multifilament

Multifilament sutures can be braided or twisted to allow easier handling, flexibility, pliability, knot-tying qualities, and greater tensile strength. Their irregular surface incites increased tissue reactivity. The interstices and capillarity of the suture may allow the harboring of bacteria, making them less appropriate for use in a contaminated field. Examples of common multifilament sutures include polyglactin 910 (Vicryl, Ethicon, Inc.), silk, and polyester (Ethibond, Ethicon, Inc.).

9.5 Suture Degradation

Suture materials are classified as absorbable or nonabsorbable to reflect the rapidity of their in vivo degradation potential. Both absorbable and nonabsorbable sutures can be further categorized by their respective configurations, reactivity, memory, or handling (Table 9.2).

Table 9.2 Physical characteristics of suture materials

Suture materials	Biochemical properties	Strength retention profile	Physical properties	Materials
Plain gut	Low tensile strength High tissue reactivity	7–10 days	Twisted monofilament	Submucosa of sheep intestine or serosa of beef intestine
Chromic gut	High tissue reactivity Treated with chromium salt to slow degradation	10–14 days	Twisted monofilament	
Vicryl (Polyglactin 910)	Easy to handle Good knot security High coefficient of friction Moderate tissue reactivity	50% at 21 days	Multifilament	Copolymer of lactide and glycolide
Monocryl (*poliglecaprone 25*)	Moderate handling Low tissue reactivity Low coefficient of friction	50% at 7 days	Monofilament	Copolymers of glycolide and ε-caprolactone
PDS II (*polydioxanone*)	High and prolonged tensile strength Low coefficient of friction Low tissue reactivity	50% at 4 weeks	Monofilament	Polyester of poly (p-dioxanone)
Silk	Good knot security Easy to handle High tissue reactivity High coefficient of friction High capillarity	Permanent[a]	Multifilament braided	Raw silk spun by silkworm

(continued)

Table 9.2 (continued)

Suture materials	Biochemical properties	Strength retention profile	Physical properties	Materials
Nylon	Poor knot security Low tissue reactivity Low coefficient of friction High degree of memory	Permanent[b]	Available in both mono- and multifilament braided configurations	Polyamide polymer
Prolene	Poor knot security Low tissue reactivity Low coefficient of friction High degree of memory	Permanent	Monofilament	Polymer of propylene
Polyester	Good knot security Easy to handle High coefficient of friction	Permanent	Multifilament braided	Polymer of polyethylene Terephthalate

[a] Loses all or most of its tensile strength at 1 year
[b] Loses 15–20% of tensile strength per year via hydrolysis

9.5.1 Absorbable

Absorbable sutures are derived from either mammalian collagen or synthetic polymers; sutures derived from mammalian collagen are degraded by proteolytic enzymes, while synthetic absorbable sutures are degraded by hydrolytic processes.

Collagen-derived sutures are made from either the submucosal layer of sheep intestines or the serosal layer of bovine intestines. The collagenous tissue is then treated with an aldehyde solution that serves to cross-link and strengthen the suture to make it more resistant to degradation. In general, collagen-based sutures are more reactive than synthetic absorbable sutures. Ideally, an absorbable suture maintains its tensile strength during the critical stages of wound healing and undergoes absorption only after sufficient tissue strength has been restored.

9.5.2 Nonabsorbable

Nonabsorbable suture materials are manufactured to resist biochemical breakdown and are designed to either persist indefinitely within the wound bed or undergo a planned later removal. Nonabsorbable sutures may be selected when prolonged tension (e.g., fascial closure or tendon repair) is anticipated or required for suitable healing to take place. Nonabsorbable suture materials, because they incite less tissue inflammation, are used in situations where scar cosmesis is prioritized – such as when suturing the skin of the face.

9.5.3 Materials

9.5.3.1 Absorbable Suture Materials

9.5.3.1.1 Plain Gut

Plain gut, also known as catgut or surgical gut, is formed from processed strands of highly purified collagen from the small intestine of sheep or cattle. The collagenous tissue is initially treated with an aldehyde solution to make it more resistant to degradation. Plain gut undergoes proteolytic degradation, and infection may accelerate the rate of suture breakdown.

There are different formulations of gut sutures that dictate their rate of absorption. The plain gut suture has a tensile strength that is maintained for only 7–10 days, with complete absorption occurring within 70 days. The plain gut can be heat-treated (generating a fast-absorbing gut) to accelerate the loss of tensile strength and absorption. This fast-absorbing gut is used primarily for epidermal suturing where sutures are required for only 5–7 days. Many plastic surgeons find this suture type useful for repairing traumatic lacerations of the face, particularly in pediatric patients who will not tolerate suture removal or in adult patients who are unlikely to follow up. Additionally, a plain gut is useful to patch any incisional gaps that may arise following a subcuticular closure. In doing so, healing by secondary intention and incisional oozing is limited.

9.5.3.1.2 Chromic Gut

The chromic gut is also collagen derived and prepared from the small intestine of sheep or cattle. Chromic gut is characteristically packaged in an alcohol-based solution and treated with salt to resist degradation The suture loses approximately 50% of its tensile strength 10–14 days following implantation, and complete resorption takes approximately 90 days. It is frequently used for intraoral and intranasal mucosal repairs. An occasional patient can develop an allergic reaction to chromic salts.

9.5.3.1.3 Vicryl (Polyglactin 910)

Polyglactin 910 (Vicryl, Ethicon, Inc.) is a synthetic, braided suture consisting of a copolymer of lactide and glycolide. It is coated with polyglactin 370 and calcium stearate to provide excellent handling and smooth rundown properties. As of 2003, a broad-spectrum antibacterial agent, triclosan, has been added (creating Vicryl Plus™, Ethicon, Inc.).

Polyglactin 910 is broken down by hydrolysis. It elicits a less vigorous tissue reaction than a plain gut suture. Animal studies indicate that the suture retains approximately 75% of its original tensile strength at 2 weeks and approximately 50% at 3 weeks for sizes 6-0 and larger. By 4 weeks, approximately 25% of the original strength is retained. All original tensile strength is lost by 5 weeks, and absorption is complete between 56 and 70 days. In plastic surgery, polyglactin 910 is most often used for soft tissue approximation.

9.5.3.1.4 Monocryl (Poliglecaprone 25)

Poliglecaprone 25 (Monocryl, Ethicon, Inc.) is a synthetic, monofilament suture comprised of copolymers of glycolide and ε-caprolactone. Poliglecaprone 25 features superior pliability for easy handling while exhibiting minimal tissue drag. It is frequently used for soft tissue closure as it is virtually inert and exhibits a predictable absorption profile. Many surgeons will select a poliglecaprone 25 suture for deep dermal and subcuticular closures, particularly in breast and body contouring procedures.

At 7 days, a poliglecaprone 25 suture retains approximately 50–60% of its original strength and approximately 20–30% at 14 days. The original tensile strength of undyed Monocryl is lost by 21 days postimplantation.

9.5.3.1.5 PDS (Polydioxanone)

Composed of the polyester poly (p-dioxanone), polydioxanone (PDS II, Ethicon, Inc.) is a synthetic monofilament suture with extended absorption and wound support for up to 6 weeks. Polydioxanone is stiffer than polyglactin 910, and its knots may become palpable or extrude if placed intradermally in thin-skinned patients.

PDS is absorbed in vivo through hydrolysis. Approximately 70% of its tensile strength remains 2 weeks postimplantation, 50% at 4 weeks, and 25% at 6 weeks. Polydioxanone is well suited for many types of soft tissue approximation.

9.5.3.2 Nonabsorbable Suture Materials

9.5.3.2.1 Silk

Silk is a braided, dyed suture made from natural fibers spun by silkworm larvae. It is coated with wax or silicone to reduce capillarity and increase surface lubrication, which provides improved handling, ease of passage through tissue, and knot rundown properties. Although classified as nonabsorbable, silk does display some amount of degradation over time.

Surgeons appreciate the excellent handling and tying qualities of silk. Unfortunately, its braided nature and capillarity predispose it to surface debris and bacterial accumulation, resulting in acute inflammation. Another known disadvantage of surgical silk is its low tensile strength compared to other available alternatives.

9.5.3.2.2 Nylon

Nylon is composed of polyamide polymers available in both mono- and multifilament configurations. It was the first synthetic suture to be introduced. The monofilament variety (Ethilon™, Ethicon, Inc.), because of its strength and nonreactivity, is used for cutaneous wound closures. While traditionally dyed black to enhance visibility, an undyed (clear) nylon suture is available to place permanently buried, deep dermal sutures.

The multifilament braided forms (Nurolon™, Ethicon, Inc., Surgilon™, and Covidien) possess similar handling qualities and knot configurations to silk sutures. However, the potential for infection with the braided form has limited its widespread adoption.

9.5.3.2.3 Prolene (Polypropylene)

Polypropylene (Prolene, Ethicon, Inc.), a linear polypropylene polymer, is a monofilament suture material whose tissue reactivity and strength are similar to monofilament nylon. The material's low coefficient of friction facilitates knot rundown and eases passage through tissue, making it ideal for use in pull-out continuous intradermal and percutaneous suture closure. Polypropylene's slipperiness comes at the cost of requiring the surgeon to place more knots for security.

Polypropylene is also known for its plasticity. As such, when postsurgical swelling occurs, the suture is able to stretch to accommodate the wound and limit tissue cut-through. However, when the swelling recedes, the suture is likely to be loose, and gapping of the wound may result. Within plastic surgery, polypropylene is commonly utilized in facial cutaneous closures where aesthetic outcomes are prioritized and in high-tension wounds that are predisposed to swelling and edema (e.g., extremity and spinal wound closures). Polypropylene sutures have been found to retain their tensile strength for up to 2 years, as opposed to nylon, which displays some element of material breakdown.

9.5.3.2.4 Polyester

Ethibond (Ethicon, Inc.) is a nonabsorbable, braided polyester suture composed of long-chain, linear polyesters. It was manufactured to provide the same high tensile strength and low tissue reactivity as the monofilament alternatives but with improved handling qualities and knot security due to its braided configuration.

Polyester suture elicits a minimal acute inflammatory reaction in the tissue, followed by a gradual encapsulation of the suture by fibrous connective tissue. Similar to polypropylene, there is no meaningful decline in polyester sutures' strength over time. Polyester sutures are used for tendon repairs and in situations where prolonged tension at a closure site is anticipated. Ethibond Excel™ is available in braided green and undyed (white) forms.

9.6 Barbed Sutures

A barbed suture is a type of knotless surgical suture that has barbs on its surface. While suturing tissue, these barbs penetrate inside the tissue and lock them into place, eliminating the need for knots to tie the suture. In some barbed sutures, the barbs are created by cuts through the thread rather than adding the barb to the suture core, which reduces the original tensile strength of the suture by reducing its functional diameter. Therefore, a larger suture size should be considered routinely. The clinical advantages of barbed sutures include reduced suturing time and reduced overall operating time. Figure 9.1 illustrates the surface of a barbed suture.

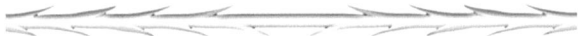

Fig. 9.1 Illustration of the surface of barbed sutures

9.7 Topical Skin Adhesives

Skin adhesives made of cyanoacrylate derivatives are useful for the closure of low-tension wounds. These transparent materials form a flexible bond over nonuniform surfaces that create a protective seal and occlusive dressing.

9.8 Needles

Surgical needles are designed to precisely thread the attached suture material through tissue while minimizing collateral injury. To do this effectively, the needle must be sharp enough to penetrate tissue with minimal resistance, rigid enough to resist bending, and flexible enough to bend before breaking. Needle performance is also influenced by the stability of the needle in the grasp of a needle holder, which is intimately related to the geometry of the needle body. As such, the overall needle architecture is also an important factor to consider when approaching wound closure. In general, today's surgical needles are produced from stainless steel alloys and contain three basic components: swage, body, and point.

9.8.1 Suture Attachment: Needle Eye/Swage

Sutures are attached to the end of the needle in two ways: eyed or swaged. A closed-eye needle has either a round, oblong, or square opening. A French split (spring design) has a split from inside the eye to the end of the needle with ridges that hold the suture in place. Eyed sutures have the disadvantage of threading and passing two strands of sutures through each hole. Swaged needles during manufacturing have the sutures placed within an opening created in the needle's end, and the swage is then crimped around the suture, securing it in place. This creates a strong attachment that prevents the surgeon from detaching the needle during multiple suturing cycles. The attached single suture avoids the time of threading and limits tissue damage. Pop-off sutures have a crimping force that is much lower and allows the surgeon to detach the suture from the needle.

9.8.2 Body

The body constitutes the majority of the needle and is the portion that is grasped by the needle holder. The body diameter should be as close as possible to the diameter of the needle. The body is designed in a variety of shapes, each with different characteristics and potential uses.

9.8.2.1 Needle Body Curvature (Fig. 9.2)

Curved needles are generally more popular because they require less space for maneuvering, but the curve must be facilitated by needle holder manipulation. The curvature may be a quarter, three-eighths, one-half, or five-eighths of a circle. The three-eighths circle requires a large arc of manipulation in deep cavities, making it preferred for large superficial wound closures, where slight wrist pronation greatly aids the surgeon. The half-circle, designed for confined spaces, requires the pronation and supination of the wrist for maneuverability. The tip can still be obscured at a depth, so the five-eighths circle needle is often better in this situation, especially for intraoral and certain urogenital and anal procedures.

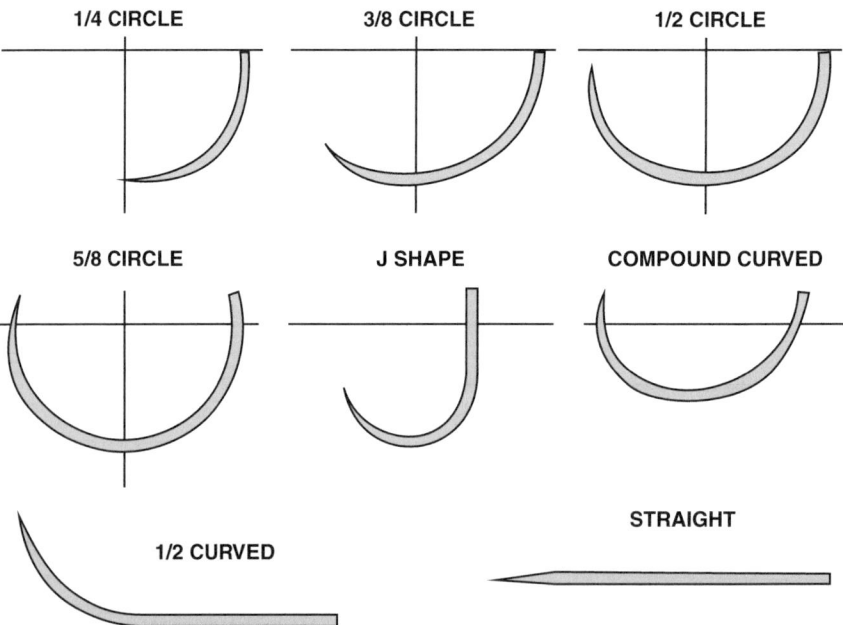

Fig. 9.2 Needle curvatures

9.8.2.1.1 Typical Uses of Needle Body Curvatures (Adapted from Byrne and Ally)

1. **Quarter-circle** short needles are useful for delicate work in superficial tissues with minimal thickness, such as eyelids and microsurgical procedures.
2. **Three-eighths circle** curved needles require smaller space for maneuvering in a confined surgical field of superficial thicker tissues. General uses include the suturing of fascia and nerves in hand surgery.
3. **One-half circle** needles require a large arc of manipulation for the needle tip to emerge if used in deep tissues. General uses for thicker tissues are used for the trunk and abdominal skin, muscle, and peritoneum.
4. **Five-eighths circle** needles are used in confined spaces and depend on a surgeon's wrist maneuverability. They are used in deeper wounds working in cavities, such as intraoral, urogenital, and anorectal procedures.
5. **J-shape** needles close deep, short incisions safely and easily. The rounded portion pushes into laparoscopic incisions safely without inadvertent visceral injury. The curved tip takes a bite of tissue on the withdrawal of the needle during laparoscopic surgery.
6. **Compound curved** has a tight 80° curvature at the tip, which is followed by a 45° curvature throughout the remainder of the body. It permits short, deep reproducible bites, with the remaining portion of the needle body forcing the needle out. It everts the wounds edges, ensuring equidistant suture placement on both sides of the incision. It is used in ophthalmic surgery for the anterior segment.
7. **One-half curved** needles are used in situations of limited exposure or space, such as movement through trocars in laparoscopic surgery or certain skin closures.
8. **Straight** needles allow direct manipulation with precision. They are ideal for use in easily accessible tissues in less-confined surgical fields.

9.8.3 Needle Point

The *point* of the needle extends from the tip to the area of the maximum cross section of the body. Each point is individually designed to the required degree of sharpness to smoothly penetrate specific tissue types. In general, there are needles with cutting edges and taper points or some that have a combination of both.

9.8.3.1 Cutting Needles

Cutting needles have at least two opposing edges that are designed to penetrate tough tissue, such as dermal tissue.

When cutting needles have three cutting edges, the position of the third cutting edge signifies whether the needle is a conventional cutting-edge needle or a reverse

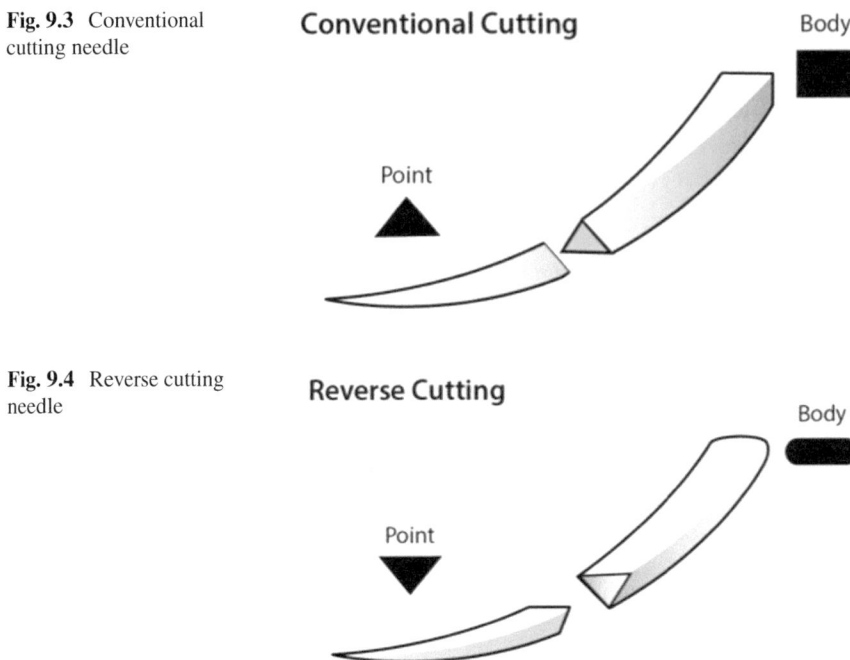

Fig. 9.3 Conventional cutting needle

Fig. 9.4 Reverse cutting needle

cutting-edge needle. In the conventional cutting needle, the third cutting edge is located on the inside, concave surface of the needle (Fig. 9.3).

Due to its location, the inside cutting edge can create a weak point in the tissue nearest to the wound edge, predisposing to suture pull-through when the necessary forces are exerted to achieve tissue apposition. In contrast, the third cutting edge of a reverse cutting-edge needle is located on the outer, convex curvature of the needle (Fig. 9.4).

When the reverse cutting needle cuts through the skin, it leaves a sufficient wall of tissue near the wound margin, against which the suture exerts its wound closure force. This wall of tissue is more likely to resist suture pull-through. Both types of cutting needles are ideal for penetrating tough tissue such as skin, which is their most common use in plastic surgery.

9.8.3.2 Taper

The taper (round) point needle has a sharp point with no sharp edge on its body, allowing for tissue spread rather than cutting (Fig. 9.5).

For this reason, the suture material is much less likely to pull through a tissue tract created by a taper needle. The point geometry and sharpness of the taper needle can be expressed by its *taper ratio*, defined as the length of the tapered portion of the needle divided by its diameter. Taper ratios typically vary from 12:1 to 8:1, with a higher ratio indicating a sharper tip. Taper point needles are recommended when

Fig. 9.5 Design of a taper tip needle

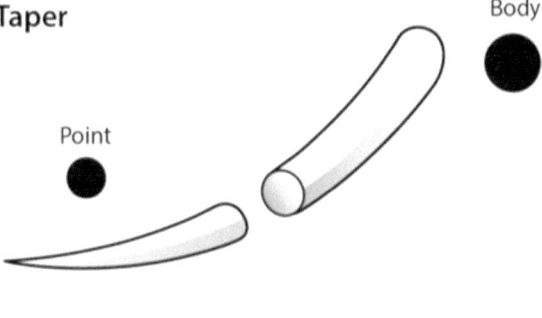

Fig. 9.6 Holding the needle on the needle holder

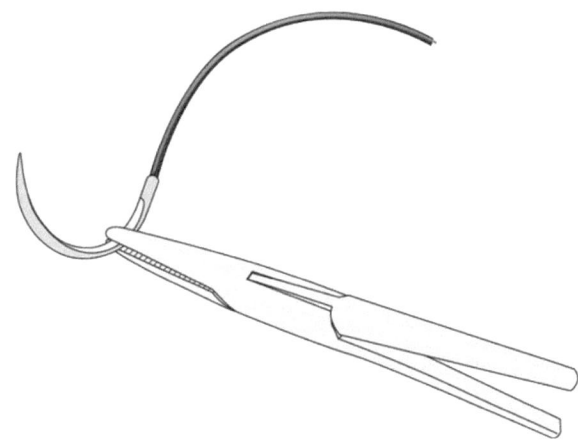

the surgeon wants to create the smallest hole possible and minimize the risk of suture pull-through. Taper point needles are appropriate for suturing cartilage, fascia, and the biliary tract.

9.8.3.3 Blunt Point Needles

Blunt point needles dissect friable tissue rather than cut it. They have a taper body with a rounded, blunt point that will not cut through tissue. They may be used for suturing the liver and kidney. Due to safety considerations, surgeons also use blunt point needles in obstetric and gynecologic procedures when working in deep cavities which are prone to space and visibility limitations.

9.8.4 Securing the Needle

Needle holders are used to pass a curved needle through tissue. Needle holder jaws may be short or flat, concave or convex, or smooth or serrated. Most needle holders have a ratchet lock. The needle holder should purchase the body away from the swage at a length of 1/3 the total distance of the body (Fig. 9.6).

A needle holder must be appropriate for the size of the needle selected. A very small needle should be held with small fine jaws. The larger and heavier the needle is, the wider and heavier the jaws of the needle holder should be. The needle holder should be the appropriate size for the procedure. If the surgeon is working deep inside the body cavity, a longer needle holder is appropriate.

Part VI
Surgical Devices

Chapter 10
Local Anesthetics

Seth Fruge and Michael Yaremchuk

10.1 Local Anesthetics

10.1.1 Mechanism of Action

Local anesthetics interrupt nerve conduction by inhibiting sodium channels [1]. In most cases, this follows their diffusion through the epineurium (connective tissue around nerves) and the neural membrane.

10.1.2 Structure

The structure of the local anesthetic molecule is also important as each component is responsible for the intrinsic properties of the local anesthetic. The molecules consist of three components: (a) lipophilic (hydrophobic) aromatic ring, (b) intermediate ester or amide chain, and (c) terminal amine (Fig. 10.1).

S. Fruge
Harvard Mass General Brigham Plastic Surgery Residency Program, Boston, MA, USA

M. Yaremchuk (✉)
Division of Plastic Surgery, Massachusetts General Hospital, and The Boston Center for Ambulatory Surgery, Inc., Boston, MA, USA
e-mail: dr.y@dryaremchuk.com

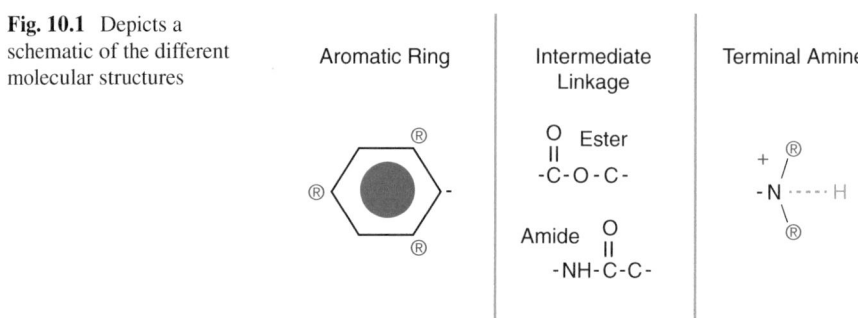

Fig. 10.1 Depicts a schematic of the different molecular structures

Table 10.1 Common local anesthetic levels of action (with and without epinephrine)

Drug class	Local anesthetic	pKa	Onset	Maximum dose without epinephrine (mg/kg)	Maximum dose with epinephrine (mg/kg)	Duration of action without epinephrine (h)	Duration of action with epinephrine (h)
Ester	Procaine	8.9	Rapid	8	10	0.75	1.5
	Tetracaine	8.5	Slow	1.5	2.5	3	10
Amide	Lidocaine	7.9	Rapid	4	7	2	4
	Mepivacaine	7.6	Medium	4	7	3	6
	Ropivacaine	8.1	Medium	2	3	3	6
	Bupivacaine	8.1	Slow	2.5	3	4	8
	Exparel	8.1	Slow	4	n/a	48–72	48–72

10.1.2.1 Onset of Action

The most important part of the local anesthetic is its terminal amine; it can exist as an ionized (H+ bound to the molecule) or a nonionized form, depending on the pH of the environment and the pKa of the local anesthetic itself. Only the nonionized (lipid-soluble) form can cross the plasma membrane of a nerve cell, where it acts to prevent a nerve from conducting a signal. This acts as the overall "on-off" switch for local anesthetics and will determine the time for the onset of action.

The *time for onset* of local anesthesia is dependent on the number of molecules that convert to the nonionized (lipid-soluble) structure when exposed to the physiologic pH (7.4) of the tissue. This is important to understand because when injecting into infected tissue, for example, the pH of the local environment is much lower than 7.4 and will further decrease the amount of nonionized local anesthetic present. In these situations, bupivacaine (pKa 8.1) would be least effective and mepivacaine (pKa 7.6) would be most likely to provide effective anesthesia. Sodium bicarbonate can also be added to the solution to increase the pH and therefore decrease the time of onset. See Table 10.1 below for the pKas of common local anesthetics and their onset of action (separated into amides and esters).

10.1.3 Potency

The aromatic ring of the local anesthetic molecule improves the lipid solubility of the compound. Lipid solubility enhances diffusion through nerve sheaths, as well as the neural membranes, as discussed above. This property correlates with *potency* because a greater portion of an administered dose can enter neurons. For example, bupivacaine is more lipid soluble than lidocaine; therefore, it is more potent and is prepared at a 0.5% concentration (5 mg/mL) rather than a 2% concentration (20 mg/mL).

10.1.4 Types of Local Anesthetics

There are two groups of local anesthetics: amides and esters. The esters are much more allergenic compared to the amides due to the fact that they are broken down into antigenic para-aminobenzoic acid (PABA). Esters are also more rapidly metabolized and less likely to cause systemic toxicity but generally have a slower onset of action due to their higher pKa.

10.1.5 Duration of Action (DOA)

The two most common local anesthetics used in plastic surgery include lidocaine (DOA: 2 h; 4 h with epinephrine) and bupivacaine (DOA: 4 h; 8 h with epinephrine). The addition of epinephrine to the local anesthetic will cause vasoconstriction to the surrounding blood vessels and reduce the ability of the local anesthetic to enter the bloodstream and disperse. This will not only increase the duration of action but will also decrease the risk of systemic toxicity. A decrease in pH will decrease the affinity of anesthetics for protein and not only decrease their efficacy but also increase the risk of systemic toxicity. Finally, a liposomal construct variant is available that dramatically increases the duration of action (Table 10.1).

10.1.6 Types of Nerve Fibers and Their Sequence of Blockade

Small fiber nerves and nerves with a higher firing rate are the first to be affected. Pain and sensory fibers are the most sensitive as they fall into this category. Nerves that are more heavily myelinated are also easier to block than unmyelinated fibers.

The sequence of blockage that a local anesthetic will follow is important to understand as this will come into play when considering the addition of epinephrine to a local anesthetic. The following list contains the order of progression of this blockade:

1. The first fibers to be blocked when injecting local anesthetic are B fibers, which have a vasodilatory effect and therefore will increase bleeding in the area (all local anesthetics have this effect, with the exception of cocaine, which has an intrinsic vasoconstrictive property).
2. The second fibers to be blocked are the C and A-delta fibers. These two fibers are responsible for pain and temperature sensation.
3. The third fiber blocked is the A-beta fibers, which are responsible for light touch and pressure sensation.
4. The last fibers to be blocked are the A-alpha and A-gamma fibers, which are responsible for motor and proprioception, respectively.

10.2 Local Anesthesia and Hemostasis

10.2.1 Vasoconstrictors and Hemostasis

Epinephrine is the most commonly used vasoconstrictive agent added to local anesthetics. It limits surrounding vasodilation, increases the duration of action, decreases the risk of systemic toxicity, and controls local bleeding. The risks associated with systemic epinephrine include tissue hypertension, tachycardia, arrhythmias, and possible tissue ischemia.

> *Contraindications to the use of epinephrine with a local anesthetic include: finger digital blocks especially when collateral circulation is compromised (trauma, vascular disease, Reynaud's), a skin flap with limited perfusion, on the penis.*

10.2.2 Dosing

Combining different local anesthetics is often performed to take advantage of the specific properties of each local anesthetic. For example, mixing lidocaine (rapid onset, short duration of action) and bupivacaine (long duration of action) will give a rapid onset to the blockade and will also have a long-lasting effect. Mixing anesthetics also gives the additional benefit of decreasing the amount of the individual anesthetics used in a block.

10.3 Safety and Toxicity

10.3.1 Maximum Dosing

The toxicity of a local anesthetic is dependent on the ability of the local anesthetic to enter the systemic circulation [2, 3]. As mentioned above, this ability is reduced by the vasoconstrictive properties of epinephrine. Some commonly used maximum dosages include lidocaine: 4.5 mg/kg (7 mg/kg with epi) and bupivacaine: 2.5 mg/kg (3 mg/kg with epi).

To calculate the maximum dose of local anesthetic (in ml), multiply the weight of the patient (in kg) by the anesthetic being used (in ml/mg) and then multiply that by the maximum dose for that anesthetic (in mg/kg). For example, the maximum dose of 1% lidocaine without epinephrine in a 100 kg patient would be = 100 kg × 1 ml/10 mg × 4.5 mg/kg = 45 ml.

10.3.2 Toxicity

The risk of systemic toxicity is increased when epinephrine is not used at the site of local anesthetic, when an amide anesthetic is used in a patient with poor hepatic function or blood flow (congestive heart failure (CHF), cirrhosis, high-dose beta blockers), and when ester anesthetics are used in patients with pseudocholinesterase deficiency.

10.3.2.1 Central Nervous System (CNS) Toxicity

- Initially, excitation symptoms are experienced as the concentration of the anesthetic increases in the CNS. This is due to the initial blockade of inhibitory neurons. Symptoms include tinnitus (ringing of the ears), muscle twitching, light-headedness, visual disturbances, numbness of the tongue and/or lips, shivering, tremors, and extreme anxiety.
- Higher concentrations will cause the overall depression of neuronal activity in the CNS. This will present as hypotension, respiratory failure, arrhythmia, bradycardia, seizures, and coma.

10.3.2.2 Cardiovascular Toxicity

- Due to the anesthetic blockade of the sodium channels in the conduction pathway (lidocaine is also considered a class 1b antiarrhythmic), systemic toxicity can present as bradycardia, hypotension, or numerous arrhythmia.

10.3.2.3 Methemoglobinemia

- Caused by the metabolite o-toluidine (most commonly from prilocaine), toxicity presents as cyanosis, shortness of breath, changes in mental status, headache, dizziness, fatigue, or loss of consciousness.

10.3.2.4 Digital Ischemia

- Digital ischemia is most likely caused by either higher than recommended concentrations of epinephrine in the anesthetic solution or by injecting into a compromised digit (trauma, Raynaud's disease, diabetes). In general, local anesthetics with epinephrine are safe to inject into the digit. An ischemic digit will appear pale and cold and have a poor capillary refill.

10.3.2.5 Allergic Reactions

- Compared to a true allergic reaction, it is much more common that patients experience either a syncopal episode associated with the fear of an injection or cardiac palpitations attributed to epinephrine (contained in the solution or released endogenously due to the anxiety of getting the injection). True allergic reactions may present as localized erythema, edema, a rash, itching, urticaria, bronchospasm, and/or hypotension.

10.4 Management of Suspected Toxicity

The management of suspected toxicity requires a high index of suspicion and should be completed in a systems-based manner [4]. The ABCs (airway, breathing, circulation) of critical care management should first be assessed and managed as needed.

IV lipid emulsion is recommended for any suspected toxicity. Further treatment will be dependent on the specific system affected: seizures can be treated with benzodiazepines and bradycardia with atropine, and arrhythmia should be treated in accordance with advanced cardiac life support (ACLS) protocols. Epinephrine-induced digital ischemia can be treated with phentolamine and with warming.

References

1. Becker DE, Reed KL. Essentials of local anesthetic pharmacology. Anesth Prog. 2006;53(3):98–108; quiz 109-10. https://doi.org/10.2344/0003-3006(2006)53[98:EOLAP]2.0.CO;2. PMID: 17175824; PMCID: PMC1693664.

2. Sekimoto K, Tobe M, Saito S. Local anesthetic toxicity: acute and chronic management. Acute Med Surg. 2017;4(2):152–60. https://doi.org/10.1002/ams2.265. PMID: 29123854; PMCID: PMC5667269.
3. El-Boghdadly K, Pawa A, Chin KJ. Local anesthetic systemic toxicity: current perspectives. Local Reg Anesth. 2018;11:35–44. https://doi.org/10.2147/LRA.S154512. PMID: 30122981; PMCID: PMC6087022.
4. Rodgers A, Walker N, Schug S, McKee A, Kehlet H, van Zundert A, Sage D, Futter M, Saville G, Clark T, MacMahon S. Reduction of postoperative mortality and morbidity with epidural or spinal anaesthesia: results from overview of randomised trials. BMJ. 2000;321(7275):1493. https://doi.org/10.1136/bmj.321.7275.1493. PMID: 11118174; PMCID: PMC27550.

Chapter 11
Electrocautery

Michael T. Bailin and Michael Yaremchuk

11.1 Electrosurgical Unit (ESU)

An electrosurgical unit (ESU) is a generator capable of creating alternating current at a high frequency to induce heat energy capable of an array of effects. Currents are adjusted to achieve coagulation by drying out cells or to cut tissues by the vaporization of cells (Fig. 11.1).

M. T. Bailin
Department of Anesthesia, The Boston Center for Ambulatory Surgery, Boston, MA, USA

M. Yaremchuk (✉)
Division of Plastic Surgery, Massachusetts General Hospital, and The Boston Center for Ambulatory Surgery, Inc., Boston, MA, USA
e-mail: dr.y@dryaremchuk.com

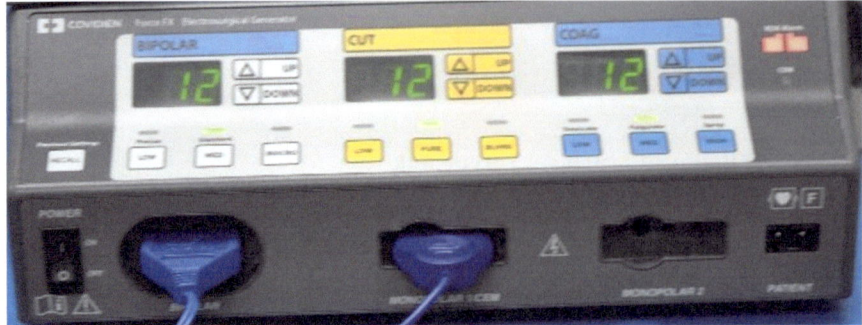

Fig. 11.1 Example of an electrosurgical unit capable of monopolar and bipolar cautery

11.2 Monopolar Electrocautery (The Bovie)

The use of high-frequency alternating electrical currents (100,000–5,000,000 Hz) to incise and coagulate tissues was developed by William T Bovie, an inventor and biophysicist. His unit was popularized by Dr. Harvey Cushing, starting in 1926 at the Peter Bent Brigham Hospital. Dr. Cushing utilized Bovie's monopolar electrosurgical unit in over 500 neurosurgical operations prior to its widespread adoption within the surgical community. As a result, the name "Bovie" is now synonymous with the monopolar electrocautery unit.

Monopolar electrocautery has the current pass from the pen-shaped probe to the tissue and through the patient to a return pad to complete the electric current circuit [1]. The return pad, or dispersive electrode, has a relatively large surface area, which is positioned on the patient. This allows high-frequency current to flow back with a low-current intensity in order to prevent any physical effects, such as undesired burns (Fig. 11.2). The probe may have multiple interchangeable tips varying in length and tip acuity. The pen is operated by pressing one of two buttons—cut or coagulate—with an additional blend-cut function, which can be utilized by changing a setting on the electrosurgical generator (Fig. 11.3). The voltage can be plotted over time for each of these functions, producing a sinusoidal curve. Each curve differs in the portion of time the current is being delivered to the device while pressing the button alternating with the periods of time in which no current is being delivered.

11.2.1 Modes of Operation

Monopolar electrosurgery, therefore, has the means of delivering energy to the tissue through several modalities (modes of operation): pure cut, blended cut, desiccation (or pinpoint), and spray (or fulguration).

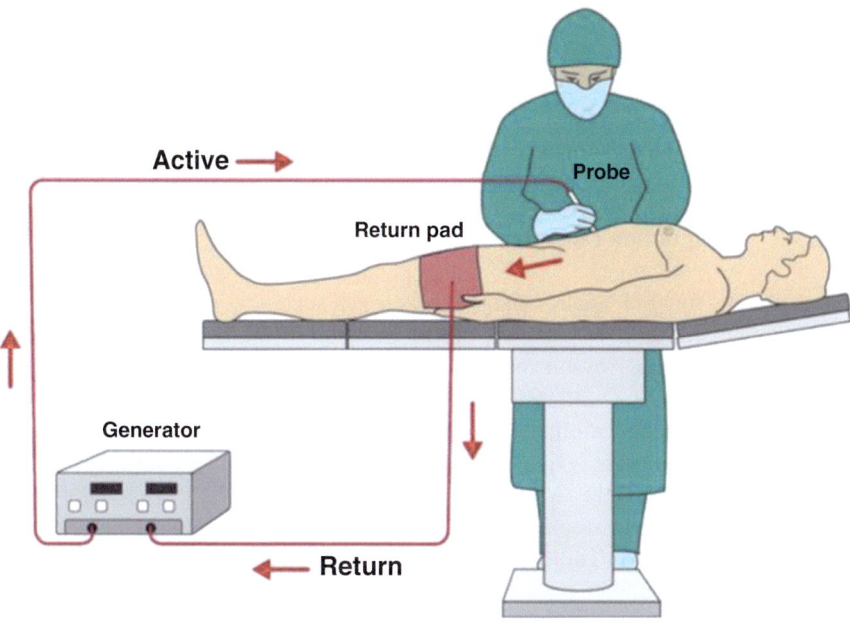

Fig. 11.2 Illustration of monopolar electrocautery circuit with the current pass from the pen-shaped probe to the tissue and through the patient to a return pad to complete the electric current circuit

Fig. 11.3 Intraoperative use of monopolar electrocautery unit

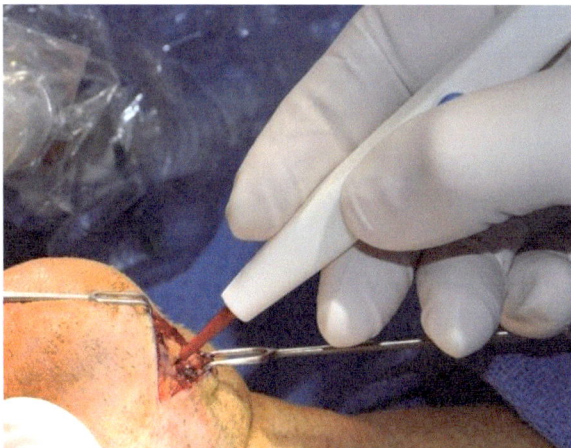

11.2.1.1 Pure Cut Function

This modality delivers moderate voltage continuously from the device tip to the involved tissue, reaching temperatures between 100° C and 400° C, resulting in the vaporization of the intracellular water and lysis of the involved cells, leaving an incision where it was aimed. The cutting effect of a monopolar ESU precedes the leading edge of the active electrode by a microscopic distance. It is the heat of the current, not the instrument that cuts. The surgeon should not apply pressure onto the tissues with the instrument but rather just guide it. The pure cut setting acts like a scalpel in that vessel are incised resulting in bleeding. There is no hemostatic effect with the incision.

11.2.1.2 Coagulation Function

The coagulate function applies electrical energy in such a way that it results in both tissue desiccation and coagulation of the proteins in the surrounding tissue, as opposed to water vaporization and cellular lysis, which occur at lower temperatures, typically between 60° C and 99° C.

There are two coagulation types, depending on the relation of the electrode to the tissue. To apply pinpoint coagulation, the surgeon holds the electrode in physical contact with or against the tissue. The tip should make only light, momentary contact with the surface to stop local bleeding. Here, an interrupted current provides controlled dehydration. The drying-out effects of a pure coagulating current produce a zone of coagulation necrosis that is limited to the surface layers of the tissue. Fulguration, or spray coagulation, is a noncontact coagulation where the current jumps or sparks from the electrode to the tissue. It is sometimes used to destroy surface layers of cells from a bed where suspicious lesions have been removed.

11.2.1.3 Blend-Cut Function

This modality allows the surgeon to cut and coagulate at the same time. The "blend-cut" function is a middle ground between cut and coagulation. There is an intermediate maximum voltage, with the current being delivered approximately 25–50% of the time the cut button is being pressed. The resulting impact on the surrounding tissue elicits both cellular lysis and the desiccation/coagulation of other cells. It is useful to resect masses of tissue and to recontour redundant tissue when cutting is continuous while allowing a minimally bloody field.

11.2.2 Monopolar Safety

The most common hazards associated with electrosurgical devices are fire, burns, and interference with electromedical devices.

11.2.2.1 Fire

The sparking and heating associated with an ESU can provide an ignition causing a fire in the operating room (OR) environment. Oxidizers such as oxygen and nitrous oxide provide a fire-friendly OR environment. They exist within the airway-ventilator circuit and in areas where open oxygen sources (e.g., nasal cannula, mask) are concentrated by the configuration of the surgical drapes. Any increase in the oxygen concentration above room air, as well as any presence of nitrous oxide, is considered oxidizer enriched. Surgical fields enhanced with oxygen markedly facilitate flammability. A standard blue towel used as a surgical drape will ignite 16 times faster (0.1 s vs. 1.6 s) in an environment of 100% oxygen (Reference [2]). There are many fuel sources that can burn in the OR. The list includes alcohol-containing prep solutions, sponges, drapes, towels, dressings, tubing, gowns, packaging materials, gastrointestinal tract gases, skin, hair, blankets, endoscopic instruments, and gloves. Supplemental oxygen (the oxidizer) is rarely required yet regularly overutilized in conscious sedation cases. Open oxygen delivery via a mask or nasal cannula is often unnecessarily applied for superficial surgical procedures on the shoulders, neck, face, and head, precisely where the drapes will concentrate excess and dangerous oxygen gas. Adding an oxidizer to complete the fire triad is a choice that should rarely be made. For patients who absolutely require supplemental oxygen (e.g., patients on home oxygen), a strong argument exists to use an airway device that will ensure no leakage of oxygen into the atmosphere (e.g., laryngeal mask or supraglottic airway).

11.2.2.2 Burns

Burn injury may result from operator error, faulty insulation of electrodes or surgical instruments, improper ESU setting, and improper placement of the grounding pad [3].

Burn injury may occur if the electrode mistakenly contacts a nearby unintended tissue due to surgical error. When using the Bovie near metal instruments, such as retractors, it is important to keep an appropriate distance from the object and to eliminate contact with the skin as the electrical current can arc to the instrument and cause thermal injury to the adjacent skin despite the presence of a grounding pad.

Instruments such as small retractors used near the area of ESU coagulation should be insulated. The integrity of such instruments should be part of the scrub nurse's overall presurgical assessment of instruments intended for the operation. A metal instrument can transfer the heat of the electrode to tissues in contact with the instrument, resulting in burn injury.

11.2.2.3 Jewelry

Removing jewelry from patients seems to be the safest practice, obviating a possible alternative return path for the current generated by the electrosurgical unit. Unintended and undesirable burns will occur if electrical energy converges around metal jewelry. As electrons follow the path of least resistance, ESU current preferentially will exit the body through a properly functioning grounding pad (dispersive electrode).

In situations where jewelry cannot be removed, or the patient refuses, several precautions should be taken. By its nature, elective surgery does not have to be

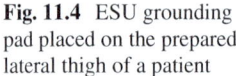
Fig. 11.4 ESU grounding pad placed on the prepared lateral thigh of a patient

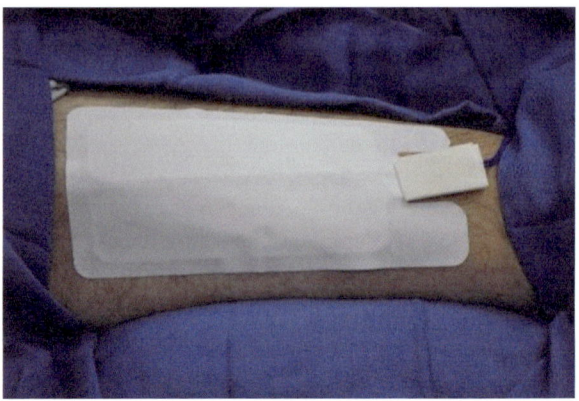

performed, but the patient and operative team may choose to proceed following additional safeguards regarding body art. Specific informed consent regarding the risk of injury, disfiguring burn, loss, or dislodgement should be included in the preoperative discussion, along with written acknowledgment (informed consent). Intraoperatively, frequent visual monitoring of metallic jewelry should be performed if possible. Other theoretically advantageous maneuvers include an attempt to insulate jewelry, using only short bursts of electrocautery, and ensuring the dispersive electrode is optimally placed (closer to the incision and further from metallic objects).

When oral, genital, or skin piercings with a tenuous tract are removed, care must be taken to preserve the channel with replacement plastic jewelry, a nonmetallic suture, or a plastic stent. Besides burn injury, complications resulting from wearing metallic jewelry during surgery include aspiration, infection, loosening, loss, pressure necrosis, and neurovascular compromise. In many centers, wedding bands are permitted on a case-by-case basis and insulated from the ground with circumferential tape. However, if the patient develops edema from fluid administration or vasodilation, the finger distal to the ring may suffer. The strongest recommendation is to ask patients to leave metal jewelry at home and obviate any possible risk of iatrogenic injury.

As the grounding pad is responsible for safely returning current to the electrosurgical generator, it provides safety via a path of low resistance and low current. The risk of burn is increased when contact quality between the patient and the grounding pad is poor. This can occur if the grounding pad is placed against an unshaven area, an area covered with moisturizers, a bony prominence, scar tissue, or an area with little soft-tissue mass. For that reason, contact area grounding pads should be positioned over dry, shaven, and well-vascularized tissue surfaces (Fig. 11.4).

11.2.2.4 Pacemaker and Internal Cardiac Defibrillator (ICD) Interference

Cardiac implantable electronic devices (CIED) have become commonplace and include implantable cardiac defibrillators/cardioverters (ICDs) and permanent pacemakers (PPMs). With advances in microcircuitry and battery technology, developments in cutting-edge devices, including lead-less PPMs and subcutaneous ICDs, are becoming more prevalent in surgical patients. Electromagnetic interference (EMI) caused by monopolar electrocautery, especially if it is within 6 in. of the pulse generator, can cause malfunctioning of the CIED. In the event of surgery above the umbilicus, reprogramming or magnet application may be necessary [4].

Although these devices possess effective algorithms to filter background noise and process physiological signals, they can and do fail in spectacular and dangerous ways.

Pacemakers can falsely interpret EMI as intrinsic atrial or ventricular cardiac activity and may not trigger a paced rhythm (oversensing) for the duration of the electrosurgical unit (ESU) activation. This may result in cardiac asystole if the patient is pacemaker dependent. Additionally, if the pacer or ICD logic circuits detect what it construes as "atrial" activity from the ESU, rapid ventricular pacing may result. It is therefore important to preoperatively determine if the patient is pacemaker dependent (does not have a perfusing rhythm without pacing). In these patients, an additional method of pacing is required, and magnet application or reprogramming to convert the pacer to asynchronous mode is needed.

Magnets can be applied to convert pacemakers to asynchronous mode, to protect them from EMI, but the response to magnet application is variable. The response can be programmed; therefore, some pacemakers will have no response, and some will pace asynchronously. The magnet effect must be confirmed prior to any operative procedure when possible.

11.3 Bipolar Electrosurgery

The method uses a set of forceps as a bipolar device. The electrical current passes from one side of the forceps, through the target tissue to the other side of the forceps, then back to the generator (Fig. 11.5). The electrical current is restricted to the tissue between the forceps, therefore not requiring the use of a grounding pad (Fig. 11.6).

Because the electrosurgical current is restricted to the tissue between the arms of the forceps electrode, thereby decreasing the amount of energy scatter, bipolar

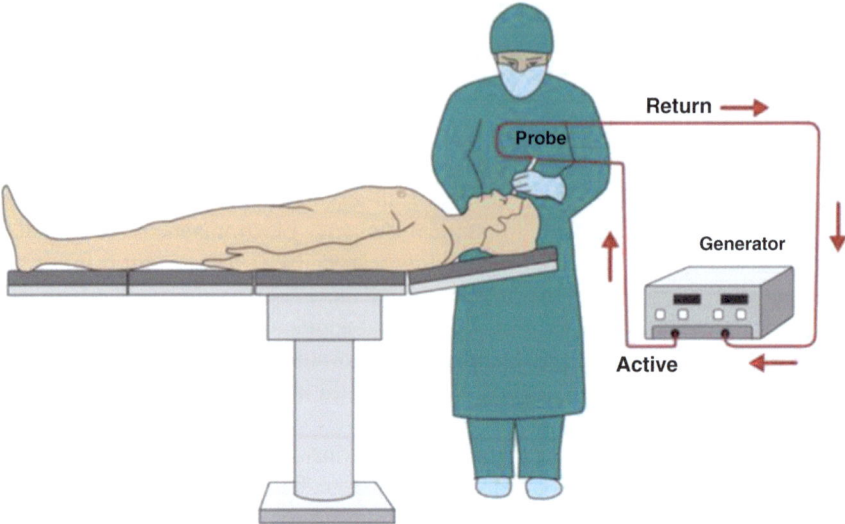

Fig. 11.5 Illustration of bipolar electrosurgery current which passes from one side of the surgeon's forceps, through the target tissue to the other side of the forceps, then back to the generator

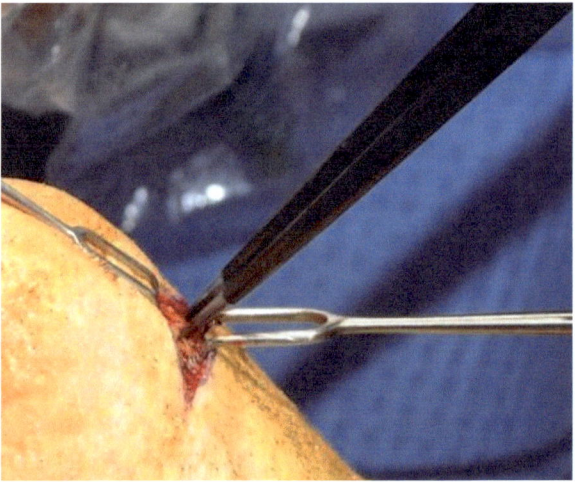

Fig. 11.6 Intraoperative use of bipolar electrosurgical unit

electrosurgery is ideal for precise cauterization of small blood vessels and nerves near vital structures.

The focal electrical current transfer of bipolar electrosurgery lessens the likelihood of fire, burns, and interference with electrosurgical devices such as pacemakers and ICDs. For patients with a CIED, where only bipolar electrosurgical current is planned, consultation with their electrophysiology team is not advantageous.

References

1. McCauley G. Understanding electrosurgery. Bovie Med Corp. 2010;4:4–15. www.boviemed.com.
2. Culp WC Jr, Kimbrough BA, Luna S. Flammability of surgical drapes and materials in varying concentrations of oxygen. Anesthesiology. 2013;119(4):770–6. https://doi.org/10.1097/ALN.0b013e3182a35303.
3. Mann D. Reducing the hazard of burns and bovie pads. Plast Reconstr Surg. 2000;106(4):947. https://doi.org/10.1097/00006534-200009040-00044.
4. Crossley GH, Poole JE, Rozner MA, Asirvatham SJ, Cheng A, Chung MK, Ferguson TB Jr, Gallagher JD, Gold MR, Hoyt RH, Irefin S, Kusumoto FM, Moorman LP, Thompson A. The Heart Rhythm Society (HRS)/American Society of Anesthesiologists (ASA) expert consensus statement on the perioperative management of patients with implantable defibrillators, pacemakers and arrhythmia monitors: facilities and patient management this document was developed as a joint project with the American Society of Anesthesiologists (ASA), and in collaboration with the American Heart Association (AHA), and the Society of Thoracic Surgeons (STS). Heart Rhythm. 2011;8(7):1114–54. https://doi.org/10.1016/j.hrthm.2010.12.023.

Chapter 12
Surgical Tourniquets

David Mattos, Brent B. Pickrell, and Michael Yaremchuk

12.1 Use of Tourniquets

In general, tourniquet use requires exsanguination of the extremity, followed by compression with the tourniquet itself to occlude blood flow into and out of the selected extremity [1, 2]. The most effective method of exsanguination involves elevation and compression of the extremity with an Esmarch bandage, named after Friedrich von Esmarch, who originally designed the device. The Esmarch bandage is an elastic rubber bandage that is used to compress the venous blood out of an extremity before activating the tourniquet, which occludes arterial inflow and venous outflow at the location where it is applied. Tourniquets can therefore only be effective distal to their sites of application; they are only useful for surgical procedures distal to the mid-thigh or mid-upper arm. While tourniquets are commonly applied before the surgical prep and drape for surgery, if the site of the operation is

---

Supplementary Information The online version contains supplementary material available at https://doi.org/10.1007/978-3-031-30835-2_12.

D. Mattos
Harvard Mass General Brigham, Boston, MA, USA
e-mail: DMATTOS1@PARTNERS.ORG

B. B. Pickrell
Harvard Mass General Brigham Plastic Surgery Residency Program, Boston, MA, USA
e-mail: BPICKRELL@PARTNERS.ORG

M. Yaremchuk (✉)
Division of Plastic Surgery, Massachusetts General Hospital, and The Boston Center for Ambulatory Surgery, Inc., Boston, MA, USA
e-mail: dr.y@dryaremchuk.com

© The Author(s), under exclusive license to Springer Nature Switzerland AG 2023
M. Yaremchuk et al. (eds.), *Expertise in the Operating Room*,
https://doi.org/10.1007/978-3-031-30835-2_12

close to the tourniquet site, a few additional centimeters of working space can be gained by applying a sterile tourniquet after first prepping and draping the patient up to the axilla or groin. The use of a sterile tourniquet also allows its removal in the event that more proximal access to the involved extremity is needed for the surgical procedure.

Pneumatic tourniquets are the safest tourniquets available today and have the lowest morbidity. Sizing is important because wider cuffs have more gradual pressure gradients from the center of the tourniquet to its edge [3]. Additionally, wide cuffs typically require lower inflation pressure to stop arterial flow. Ideally, the cuff width to limb circumference ratio should be greater than 1:2. Once applied, the tourniquet cuff should overlap itself a length of 3–6 in. Any less and the tourniquet may unexpectedly release intraoperatively. Any more may increase the rolling and wrinkling of the underlying soft tissue.

Nonpneumatic tourniquets are rarely used in hospitals today, given that they often produce tourniquet pressures that are unnecessarily higher than the limb occlusion pressure. These have higher levels of morbidity and are almost exclusively used in military settings, such as to stop arterial limb bleeding during military operations or traumas outside of the hospital.

12.2 Tourniquet Application (See Video 12.1)

Tourniquets can be placed on the upper or lower extremities. They should not be placed over joints where there is insufficient underlying soft tissue. Prior to application, a layer of soft padding (such as Webril) should be placed to prevent the shearing or damaging of the skin. For upper extremity procedures, the decision of whether to place the tourniquet on the forearm or arm depends on the operative site. For short cases, placing the tourniquet on the arm is usually easy and reliable. A nonsterile tourniquet can be placed before the prep and protected with a clear impermeable drape to prevent fluid from getting under the tourniquet. If there is a possibility that the dissection may need to extend under the area of the tourniquet, a sterile tourniquet that can be removed intraoperatively should be used. One consideration to remember is that procedures with longer tourniquet times or expected multiple tourniquet runs will lead to more ischemia and the reperfusion of metabolites if more of the extremity is ischemic under the tourniquet. A forearm tourniquet may be useful in those scenarios.

The type of anesthesia being used during a case may dictate the location of the tourniquet. When using a Bier block, where anesthetic is injected into the extremity intravenously and allowed to diffuse locally, the tourniquet acts as a barrier. It is better to use a more distal tourniquet if possible to minimize the dose of local anesthetic necessary for effect and to minimize the amount of time that the tourniquet has to be up. If the tourniquet is placed on the forearm during a Bier block, it often needs to be up for 30 min minimum to prevent systemic toxicity after it is released.

In these scenarios, especially in procedures expected to be longer than 1 h, a double cuff tourniquet can be used. This allows the diffusion of local anesthetic into the more distal cuff region and then filling of the distal cuff before releasing the proximal one to compress the anesthetized area and minimize tourniquet pain, which usually presents after 1 h.

12.3 Tourniquet Placement

After the tourniquet is placed, the extremity is exsanguinated with the use of an Esmarch bandage, except when there is a cancerous mass or infection in the involved extremity. In those circumstances, it is safer to simply elevate the extremity for a few minutes before inflating the tourniquet to avoid compressing the soft tissue surrounding the infection or cancer, which could theoretically lead to its systemic spread. The next decision is pressure setting for the tourniquet. Most often, 250 mmHg is used for the upper extremity and 300 mmHg for the lower extremity, but the value can be determined by understanding the limb occlusion pressure (LOP) concept. Originally measured manually with the use of a stethoscope, the LOP is the pressure at which an inflating tourniquet stops distal arterial flow. One should use the lowest tourniquet pressure possible to lower the risk of tourniquet-related complications. A margin of 50–100 mmHg is often added over the LOP to allow for fluctuating conditions in surgery. For practical reasons, many surgeons add a margin over a patient's systolic blood pressure.

For normotensive patients, using a tourniquet inflation pressure of 250 mL of mercury (mmHg) for the upper extremity gives the surgeon at least 100 mmHg over the patient's systolic pressure. One should remember that while correlated, the inflation pressure of the tourniquet is not the same pressure felt within the tissues and that the thicker the soft tissue layer is, the less the inflation pressure of the tourniquet transmits through the soft tissue. For this reason, lower extremity tourniquets are often set at higher temperatures (e.g., 300 mmHg). Finally, certain medical conditions that result in arterial calcification (diabetes mellitus or peripheral vascular disease) may merit additional tourniquet pressures to achieve proper arterial occlusion.

12.4 Tourniquet Guidelines

After inflating a tourniquet, the surgeon should closely monitor the inflated time. Tourniquet time produces ischemia, whose length is related to tourniquet-related complications. Two hours of tourniquet time is usually considered safe. Animal studies suggest that for up to 2 h, the functional and physiologic impacts, while measurable, are reversible. During long operations where multiple tourniquet runs are needed, a 20–30 min break for the reperfusion of the limb between tourniquet inflations is a useful, guiding timeline. One should also consider the timing of medications, particularly intravenous antibiotics, which should be given at least 5–10 min before the tourniquet is inflated to allow adequate time for tissue penetration.

12.5 Tourniquet Effects and Complications

Tourniquets cause systemic and tissue compression and ischemia. They include tourniquet pain, as well as cardiovascular, metabolic, pharmacologic, and functional effects. Possible complications include skin injury, nerve injury, muscle injury, etc [4–9].

Tourniquet pain is multifactorial and driven by the duration of use, cuff pressure, and cuff diameter. Typically, the first 30 min is well tolerated, but in awake patients, the tourniquet pain continues to worsen after 30 min. A dull, aching sensation first at the site of the tourniquet may then progress to numbness and paralysis of the extremity distal to the tourniquet site. Patients often have to be sedated further to help combat tourniquet pain at this point. The release of the tourniquet itself and reperfusion of the limb can be painful as well, sometimes worse than the pain associated with tourniquet inflation.

Cardiovascular effects are largely driven by the changes in blood volume during the exsanguination of the extremity and then deflation of the tourniquet. The exsanguination preceding tourniquet inflation increases blood volume, systemic vascular resistance, and central venous pressure. These increases persist until tourniquet deflation, when the blood volume rushes back into the extremity, dropping mean arterial pressure and central venous pressure. Tourniquet pain and ischemia after about an hour of use can also increase heart rate and blood pressure. Healthy patients tolerate these changes well, but sick patients and those with significant comorbidities are less able to cope. Cardiovascular changes upon deflation are also influenced by the redistribution of metabolites from the ischemic limb into the systemic circulation.

The metabolic changes seen after tourniquet release are caused by anaerobic metabolites that build in the ischemic limb while the tourniquet is inflated. Their release into the bloodstream contributes to hypotension, metabolic acidosis, hyperkalemia, and myoglobulinemia. In more significant cases, this can lead to myoglobinuria and renal failure, which are more likely to occur in larger limbs and with longer tourniquet inflation times. In scenarios of trauma, where a tourniquet is applied in the field and the warm ischemia time is prolonged, the treating physician should expeditiously remove the tourniquet in a controlled environment. This includes the utilization of cardiac monitors, with appropriate staff ready, such as the anesthesia team, to help treat the effects of the release of metabolites into the circulation. Metabolic derangements in settings of prolonged tourniquet time from trauma can be severe enough to cause cardiac arrest.

Functional effects are typically transient. Studies have compared surgery with and without tourniquets, such as during anterior cruciate ligament reconstruction, and have found that patients with a tourniquet had measurable electromyography (EMG) changes, increased quadriceps atrophy, and decreased strength compared to the non-tourniquet group in the first few months. The changes normalized by the time of a 1-year follow-up [10, 11].

Though uncommon, tourniquet use can cause damage to the underlying skin and soft tissues. This includes ecchymosis, damage due to shearing forces, and ischemic changes. Other complications, such as direct vascular injury, are exceedingly rare and most common in children, the elderly, and patients with peripheral vascular disease. Paresthesia and nerve injury are also rare but possible. Again, these effects can be minimized by following proper tourniquet application techniques as well as minimizing tourniquet ischemia time as much as possible.

References

1. Oragui E, Parsons A, White T, Longo UG, Khan WS. Tourniquet use in upper limb surgery. Hand (N Y). 2011;6(2):165–73.
2. Kumar K, Railton C, Tawfic Q. Tourniquet application during anesthesia: "what we need to know?". J Anaesthesiol Clin Pharmacol. 2016;32(4):424–30.
3. Younger AS, McEwen JA, Inkpen K. Wide contoured thigh cuffs and automated limb occlusion measurement allow lower tourniquet pressures. Clin Orthop Relat Res. 2004;428:286–93.
4. Pedowitz RA, Gershuni DH, Schmidt AH, Friden J, Rydevik BL, Hargens AR. Muscle injury induced beneath and distal to a pneumatic tourniquet: a quantitative animal study of effects of tourniquet pressure and duration. J Hand Surg Am. 1991;16(4):610–21.
5. Shaw JA, Murray DG. The relationship between tourniquet pressure and underlying soft-tissue pressure in the thigh. J Bone Joint Surg Am. 1982;64(8):1148–52.
6. Pedowitz RA, Gershuni DH, Friden J, Garfin SR, Rydevik BL, Hargens AR. Effects of reperfusion intervals on skeletal muscle injury beneath and distal to a pneumatic tourniquet. J Hand Surg Am. 1992;17(2):245–55.
7. Fitzgibbons PG, Digiovanni C, Hares S, Akelman E. Safe tourniquet use: a review of the evidence. J Am Acad Orthop Surg. 2012;20(5):310–9.
8. Horlocker TT, Hebl JR, Gali B, Jankowski CJ, Burkle CM, Berry DJ, et al. Anesthetic, patient, and surgical risk factors for neurologic complications after prolonged total tourniquet time during total knee arthroplasty. Anesth Analg. 2006;102(3):950–5.
9. McEwen JA. Tourniquet safety: mechanisms and prevention of injuries. 2020. https://tourniquets.org/tourniquet-injuries-mechanisms-and-prevention/.
10. Arciero RA, Scoville CR, Hayda RA, Snyder RJ. The effect of tourniquet use in anterior cruciate ligament reconstruction. A prospective, randomized study. Am J Sports Med. 1996;24(6):758–64.
11. Daniel DM, Lumkong G, Stone ML, Pedowitz RA. Effects of tourniquet use in anterior cruciate ligament reconstruction. Art Ther. 1995;11(3):307–11.

Part VII
Wound Closure

Chapter 13
Drains

Swapnil Kachare, David Straughan, and Michael Yaremchuk

13.1 Active (Suction) Drains

13.1.1 Indications

Suction drains are appropriate for clean (Class I and Class II) wounds. A Class I clean wound assumes no contamination with bacteria and usually does not involve the respiratory, alimentary, or urinary tracts. Breast implant surgery, for example, involves a Class I wound appropriate for suction drainage. These incisional wounds are surgically created and closed immediately to avoid contamination. A Class II clean-contaminated wound is similar to Class I, except for the fact that the alimentary, oropharynx, or urinary tracts are entered without a break in the sterile technique. For example, a cheek implant placed through an intraoral approach would be appropriate for use of a suction drain.

13.1.2 Function

A suction drain is a closed system that collects fluid from the body cavity and drains it into a reservoir through a pressure gradient generated by the suction bulb. The main function of these active drains is the removal of fluids (serum, blood, or

---

S. Kachare · D. Straughan
Massachusetts General Hospital and The Boston Center for Ambulatory Surgery, Inc., Boston, MA, USA

M. Yaremchuk (✉)
Division of Plastic Surgery, Massachusetts General Hospital, and The Boston Center for Ambulatory Surgery, Inc., Boston, MA, USA
e-mail: dr.y@dryaremchuk.com

© The Author(s), under exclusive license to Springer Nature Switzerland AG 2023
M. Yaremchuk et al. (eds.), *Expertise in the Operating Room*,
https://doi.org/10.1007/978-3-031-30835-2_13

lymph) to allow tissue apposition and healing [1]. The removal of serum and blood ooze allows the coaptation of tissue planes and prevents subsequent serum leak and blood ooze.

"Suction drains do not eliminate bleeding but are useful for early identification of the problem."

A suction drain prevents communication, and therefore contamination, from the outside environment.

13.1.3 Design

Suction drains are closed systems that involve perforated tubes that reside in the cavity connected to a suction reservoir outside the patient. The two most common systems vary in the design of tube perforation.

The Jackson-Pratt (JP) drain is named after Dr. Frederick Jackson and Dr. Richard Pratt, two neurosurgeons from the Naval Hospital at Camp Pendleton in California in 1971 [2]. The two surgeons were attempting to create a "brain drain," which was meant to serve as a sterile, closed system drain that could be used in craniotomy cases. The JP design is made of silicone and is oval shaped with numerous orifices and intraluminal corrugations, as shown in Fig. 13.1. The Blake drain was invented by inventor Larry Blake in 1988. This drain consists of a cylindrical silicone catheter with a solid crossed-shaped center and four open-fluted channels, also shown in Fig. 13.1. The channel as opposed to perforations is less likely to occlude with hematoma or debris.

Reservoir systems are bulbs that are collapsible and provide suction. They have plugs that allow drainage of their contents. Smaller reservoirs generate more negative pressure and therefore evacuate more fluid over a given time. Compression of the reservoir from the sides, rather than "bottom-up," generates more negative pressure within the system.

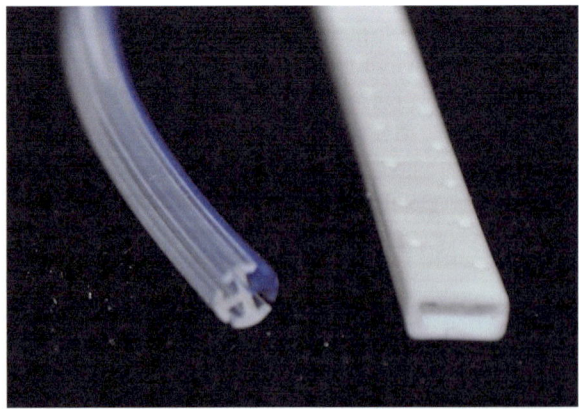

Fig. 13.1 Examples of active drains. Left—Blake (fluted), right—Jackson Pratt (perforated)

13 Drains

To dislodge a clot or debris within the tube, the tube should be routinely stripped. Stripping the tube increases negative pressure. "Stripping" involves purchasing the tube near its exit from the skin with one hand, while the other hand is compressing the tube and sliding it to the reservoir (preferably with some lubricant to decrease friction). Once the length of the drain is stripped, the end closest to the surgical site should then be released. This maneuver increases the negative pressure.

13.1.4 Skin Exit and Stabilization

Since a suction drain creates its own pressure gradient and does not depend on gravity, the drain may exit the surgical wound from the most convenient anatomic area. Considerations include patient comfort, ease of nursing care for the drain, distance from the potential cavity to the skin surface, and the presence of a foreign body. An inadequate distance of drain travel between the drainage site and the environment may contaminate the cavity, resulting in loss of suction or contamination of the surgical area. The drain should be firmly secured to the skin's surface to prevent drain migration and potential contamination.

13.1.5 Drain Removal

Based on clinical experience, the mantra for drain removal is normally a measured output of less than 20 to 30 cc for 2 consecutive days. That amount and duration assume that the drainage is now clinically insignificant. Six randomized controlled trials showed that this time-tested approach was superior to predetermined postoperative time removal with regard to decreasing seroma reaccumulation [3].

13.1.6 Antibiotics

The Centers for Disease Control and Prevention (CDC) recommends the discontinuation of antibiotics at a maximum of 24 h after a clean elective surgery [4]. The corollary is that antibiotic treatment beyond 24 hours is not indicated for the presence of suction drains. Antibiotics to avoid retrograde microbial seeding should not be used as prophylaxis for inappropriate suction drain positioning and post-op management. No evidence-based medicine supports the use of postoperative antibiotics for drains that remain in place [5, 6].

13.2 Passive Drains

13.2.1 Indications

Passive drains maintain the opening of contaminated wounds and allow the egress of their infected materials. Contaminated wounds are classified as Class III and Class IV. Class III wounds are wounds made during an operation in which major breaks in the sterile technique or gross spillage from the gastrointestinal (GI) tract occurs. Class IV wounds are infected wounds with retained devitalized tissue.

13.2.2 Design

The most common passive drain is the Penrose drain (Fig. 13.2).

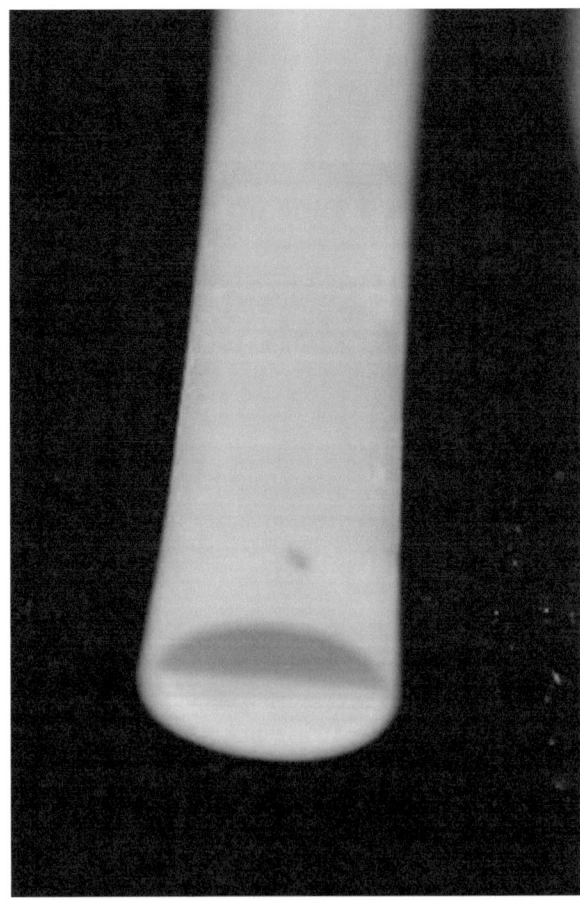

Fig. 13.2 Clinical example of a Penrose drain (smooth, passive)

The Penrose drain is a simple, hollow, rubber tube that is easily collapsible and allows fluid removal by gravity and capillarity [7]. Given its dependence on gravity and collapsibility, the Penrose drain should exit the most inferior aspect of the wound, and great care should be taken to ensure that it remains patent and in place. Since it is an open system, the drain can also be used to irrigate into the surgical cavity, with the subsequent egress of fluid via the same path.

13.2.3 Positioning

A Penrose drain is placed in the depth and remote aspect of the wound. Because drainage is dependent on gravity, it should exit at the most dependent area of the wound (Fig. 13.3).

13.2.4 Drain Removal

As the drainage subsides, a passive drain is removed sequentially. Gradual drain removal allows the area of removal to collapse and heal secondarily.

13.2.5 Skin Immobilization

Partial removal with advancement of the drain requires the need to again immobilize the drain to the skin surface. This discomfort to the patient can be avoided by creating a platform, such as a larger diameter suture tied to the skin in a way that a second suture can be used to purchase the drain and the platform (see Fig. 13.4).

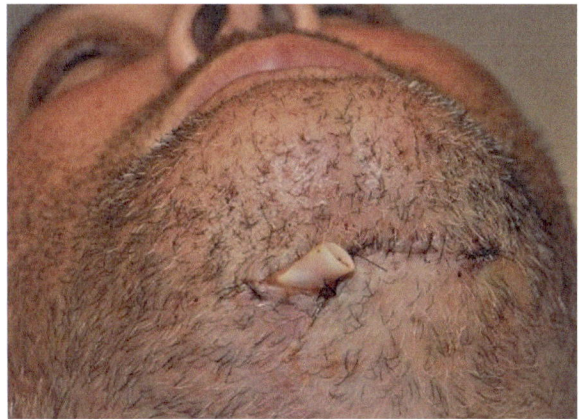

Fig. 13.3 A Penrose drain was used to drain a mandible fracture that was infected after repair. It was gradually advanced, allowing the depth of the wound to collapse

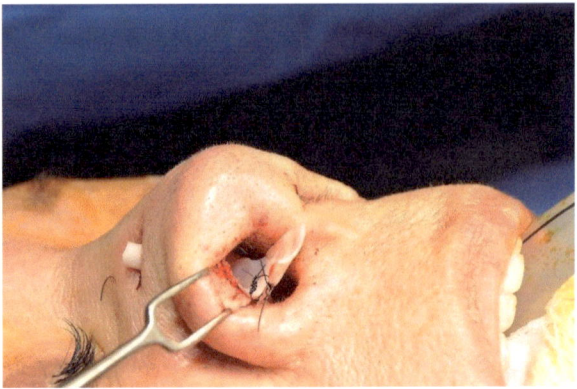

Fig. 13.4 Suture stabilization of a Penrose drain treating a traumatic nasal infection. A nylon suture was secured to the base of the nostril opening. It was tied in a way to allow a second suture to slide within the loop. The second suture then secured the passive drain. The second suture was divided to allow the advancement of the drain. The advanced drain was secured with another suture placed through the nylon suture secured to the base of the nostril opening. The passive drain was gradually advanced, allowing the depth of the wound to collapse

13.3 Summary

1. Active drains (JP (perforated) or Blake (fluted) suction drains) create their own pressure gradient. They are used in clean (Class I and Class II) surgically created closed wounds.
2. Suction drains should be positioned to avoid environmental contamination of the wound contents.
3. No evidence supports the use of antibiotics for the presence of suction drains.
4. Passive drains (e.g., Penrose) rely on gravity and capillarity for fluid evacuation. They are used for open-contaminated (Class III and Class IV) wounds.
5. Passive drains are removed sequentially to allow gradual secondary healing.
6. The use of antibiotics is appropriate for open wounds when there is evidence of active clinical infection.

References

1. Kocak E. Optimizing the closed suction drainage system. Plast Surg Nurs. 2013;33:38–42.
2. Meyerson JM. A brief history of two common surgical drains. Ann Plast Surg. 2016;77:4–5.
3. Droeser RA, Freu DM, Oertli D, et al. Volume-controlled vs no/short-term drainage after axillary lymph node dissection in breast cancer surgery, a meta-anaylsis. Breast. 2009;18(2):109–14.
4. Surgical Site Infection (SSI) Event: Center for Disease Control. 2010. http://www.cdc.gov/nhsn/PDFs/pscManual/9pscSSIcurrent.pdf?agree=yes&next=Accept. Accessed 30 Mar 2020.

5. Phillips BT, Wang ED, Mirrer J, et al. Current practice among plastic surgeons of antibiotic prophylaxis and closed-suction drains in breast reconstruction: experience, evidence, and implications for postoperative care. Ann Plast Surg. 2011;66:460–5.
6. Clayton JL, Bazakas A, Lee CN, et al. Once is not enough: withholding postoperative prophylactic antibiotics in prosthetic breast reconstruction is associated with an increased risk of infection. Plast Reconstr Surg. 2012;130(3):495–500.
7. Romm S. The persons behind the name: Charles Bingham Penrose. Plast Reconstr Surg. 1982;70:397.

Chapter 14
Suture Closure

Brent B. Pickrell and Michael Yaremchuk

14.1 Surgical Knots

A surgical knot is constructed to maintain tissue apposition during the critical early stages of wound healing. It is important that each knot be tied with precision along with the appropriate tension and orientation within the wound bed. A knot that is tied with poor technique, excess tension, or incorrect orientation may slip, incite unnecessary tissue injury, or extrude, respectively.

Proficiency in knot tying is requisite for the acquisition of all other surgical skills. For the novice (medical student or junior resident), these skills should be practiced daily to improve speed, technique, and efficiency. Not only will diligent practice improve one's hand-eye coordination, but knot tying is also one of the few surgical skills that can be reliably practiced outside of the operating room. Practicing with surgical silk (size #2–0 or #3–0) is advised, given its excellent handling properties and low cost.

Surgical knots can be tied either by hand (manual) or by instrument techniques. In hand tying, knots can be tied either one- or two-handed. There are benefits and

Supplementary Information The online version contains supplementary material available at https://doi.org/10.1007/978-3-031-30835-2_14.

B. B. Pickrell
Harvard Mass General Brigham Plastic Surgery Residency Program, Boston, MA, USA

M. Yaremchuk (✉)
Division of Plastic Surgery, Massachusetts General Hospital, and The Boston Center for Ambulatory Surgery, Inc., Boston, MA, USA
e-mail: dr.y@dryaremchuk.com

drawbacks to each technique, but the master surgeon should be proficient in each approach. Prior to discussing the different methods of knot tying, a general overview of surgical knots is provided.

14.2 Knot Construction

There are sequential steps that must be performed to construct a surgical knot [1–6]. The first step is the sequence of the formation of a *suture loop*. When one performs a standard interrupted percutaneous skin closure, this involves passing the needle perpendicularly through one wound edge, visualizing the needle-suture construct within the wound base, entering the opposing wound edge at the same tissue depth, and then passing the needle up through the skin of the opposing side equidistant from the wound edge. Bringing the hands together while grasping both suture ends will display the suture loop.

Next, the free (i.e., needle-less) suture end is wrapped around the fixed suture end (i.e., with an attached needle) and passed, either once or twice, through the suture loop to create a *throw*. After a single- or double-wrapped throw is created, it is advanced toward the wound surface. Once the throw has interfaced with the wound surface, it can be tensioned to approximate the wound edges; doing this will also provide a preview of the adequacy and aesthetics of the closure. If the wound edges do not line up satisfactorily (i.e., due to asymmetric capture of the wound edges), then the suture should be removed and the process reattempted. Applying excess tension may strangulate tissue within the suture loop and should be avoided.

A *knot* consists of two or more throws in succession. Following suture loop formation and the initial single- or double-wrapped throws, sufficient subsequent throws should be added to prevent knot unraveling (slippage); each subsequent throw should rest firmly against its predecessor. The number of throws to secure a knot is greatly dependent on the knot configuration and suture material, with non-braided monofilament sutures generally requiring a greater number of throws to ensure knot security. While too few throws can result in knot slippage, generating too many throws offers no additional knot security, and the extraneous foreign material may instead increase risks of foreign body reaction and infection or become a source of patient discomfort.

Throws can be performed in different configurations to affect the overall biomechanical performance of the knot. When two identical, consecutive single-wrapped throws are placed, a *granny knot* is constructed. This is in contradistinction to two alternating, single-wrapped throws, which produce a *square knot*, and a single double-wrapped throw followed by an alternating single-wrapped throw, which generates a *surgeon's knot*. Square and surgeon's knots have been shown to have similar overall risks of knot failure when performed correctly.

14.2.1 Slip Knots and Square Knots

14.2.1.1 The Square Knot

Although flat, square knots have long been considered the iconic surgical knot. The tying of square knots in everyday practice is often challenging and impractical. Tying a true square knot requires the application of symmetric tension to both suture ends in a straight line that is perpendicular to the axis of the knot. In a deep space or cavity, asymmetric tension applied to the suture ends is inevitable and results in the conversion of the intended square knot into two half-hitches. As such, what many surgeons consider to be square knots are in fact converted, unknowingly, to *slip knots* in vivo. One will observe that two alternating, single-wrapped (square) throws and two identical, single-wrapped (granny) throws may be easily transformed into *slip*, or *sliding*, knots by applying asymmetric tension to one suture end; however, this is not the case with the surgeon's knot.

"Many surgeons will find slip knots to be useful for the initial, preliminary approximation of wound edges subjected to significant tension."

Although an initial double-wrapped throw is also helpful to approximate tissue edges under tension, a slip knot has greater initial holding power and can be performed without needing to reverse one's hands. In practice, holding tension on one suture end during knot tying will consistently result in the formation of slip knots. Identical and nonidentical (alternating) slip knots can also be produced. Alternating slip knots are generally stronger than slip knots as they consist of nonidentical throws, and therefore they are preferred. Once there is an approximation of the wound edges, the slip knot can be converted to and finished as a square knot by using alternating, single-wrapped flat throws.

14.3 Knot Failure

Knots may fail by either slippage (unraveling) or breakage. If the surgeon fails to place an adequate number of throws, a knot is at risk of failure from slippage. Similarly, inappropriate tension and the rate of tension applied to the suture ends also influence the risk of slippage. Firm tension applied slowly to the suture ends is preferred over less tension applied rapidly. The degree of slippage also depends on the suture material (i.e., coefficient of friction) and knot technique (square versus granny).

When a knot fails by breakage, this nearly always occurs at the knot itself. As mentioned previously, the force required to break a suture material decreases once a suture is tied. As such, increasing the number of throws will necessarily weaken a given suture material.

14.4 Hand Tying

Hand tying consists of one- and two-handed methods. Two-handed knot tying is frequently the first knot-tying method introduced to medical students and is typically the easiest technique to learn and reliably reproduce. While the two-handed tie allows the operator to apply continuous tension to both ends of the suture prior to securing the knot, it is not easily performed in deep cavities, where the one-handed technique becomes favorable.

14.4.1 Two-Hand Tying

After the suture has been threaded through the wound edges, the fixed end and the free end will lie on opposite sides of the wound. For the right-handed surgeon, the fixed end is typically held in the left hand. When possible, hands should be positioned on each side of and parallel to the suture loop, which will prevent having to cross one hand over the other. Crossing one's hand is cumbersome and limits the degree of tension that can be applied. The detailed steps of the two-handed tie with the aforementioned recommended setup are outlined below and also shown in Videos 14.1 and 14.2:

Step 1: The free suture end lying on the side of the wound furthest from the operator is grasped between the tips of the right thumb and index finger, while the tips of the left thumb and index finger grasp the fixed suture end from the closer side of the wound.

Step 2: The left thumb passes underneath and then extends out against the fixed suture end so that the dorsal aspect of the thumb (i.e., nail plate) rests against the suture. If performed correctly, this should produce a backward "L" in the fixed suture end, with the remainder of the suture material resting in the left palm. The free suture end in the right hand is then laid over the proximal pulp of the left thumb so that the two suture ends are now crossed and create an "X," with the left thumb directly beneath.

Step 3: The tip of the left thumb advances up through the suture loop and meets the tip of the left index finger. Then, together as a unit, the tips of the left index finger and thumb rotate back down through the loop via wrist supination toward the body of the surgeon so that at the completion of the rotation only the left index finger remains in the loop. The left index and thumb will then encounter the free suture end that is being held by the right index finger and thumb.

Step 4: The free suture end, held by the right hand, is then grasped between the tips of the left index finger and thumb. The right hand releases the free suture end, which is then passed up through the suture loop via wrist pronation. Of technical note, one should always attempt to pass the free end rather than the fixed end with its needle through the suture loop to avoid inadvertent needle-stick injury.

Step 5: After the suture end has been passed through the suture loop, the right index finger and thumb then come around, regrasp the free suture end, and pull it through the loop. Each hand then applies perpendicular tension to its respective suture end, which advances the single-wrapped throw to the wound surface. In the setup described, the right hand is brought toward the surgeon's body to lay down a flat throw.

Step 6: To perform the second throw, the left index finger is first routed under the fixed suture end and extended out so that the dorsal aspect of the left index finger rests against the suture. With the remainder of the fixed suture end in the left hand, this will create a right angle.

Step 7: The free suture end in the right hand is then laid over the proximal pulp of the left index finger so that the two suture ends create an "X" overlying the left index finger.

Step 8: The left thumb tip then approaches and makes contact with the tip of the left index finger. Together as a unit, the tips of the left index finger and thumb rotate back down through the loop via wrist pronation away from the body of the surgeon so that at the completion of the rotation only the left thumb remains within the loop. The left index and thumb will then encounter the free suture end that is being held by the right index finger and thumb.

Step 9: The free suture end, held by the right hand, is grasped between the tips of the left index finger and thumb. The right hand then releases the free suture end, which is passed down back through the suture loop via wrist supination.

Step 10: After the suture end has been passed up through the suture loop, the right index finger and thumb come around and regrasp the free suture end and pull it through the loop. Each hand then applies perpendicular tension to its respective suture end, which advances the second single-wrapped throw to the wound surface.

14.4.2 Instrument Tying

Most plastic surgeons use instrument tying in daily practice for both percutaneous interrupted suturing and deep dermal suture placement. The instrument tie is particularly useful when one or both ends of the suture material are short and in situations where hand tying is not possible (e.g., microsurgery). This tying technique also helps conserve suture material and is advantageous when multiple operators are working simultaneously to close a sizable wound.

An instrument tie begins with the formation of suture loops over an instrument, most commonly a needle holder. Depending on the handedness of the surgeon, one hand is assigned to hold the needle holder while the other hand will manipulate the fixed suture end. After the suture has been threaded through the wound edges, the fixed suture end and the free suture end will lie on opposite sides of the wound. Ideally, the free suture end should be only a couple of centimeters in length to allow it to stand on end for easy grasping in the subsequent steps and to facilitate passage through the loops. Minimizing the length of the free suture end will also limit the motion required by the needle holder to make each throw more compact and efficient. Similarly, the hand controlling the fixed suture end should not be held out beyond 15 cm of the working area as this prohibits good control when forming the loop. The needle holder is then placed perpendicular to the line formed by the two suture ends and centered over the axis of the wound. The fixed suture end is picked up between the index finger and thumb and looped over the needle driver once or twice. Doing this will create perpendicular loops around the needle holder. Next, the needle holder should grasp the free end of the suture while remaining within the confines of the loop and pull the free end of the suture through the loop. If the intention is to create a square throw, then the free suture end should be pulled to the opposite side of the wound.

14.5 Technical Considerations for Primary Wound Closure

14.5.1 General

Precise wound closure is an important component of any operation and warrants as much consideration and planning as other key portions of the procedure. However, wound closure frequently becomes an afterthought to many surgeons, who may feel pressed for time, particularly at the end of a difficult or lengthy operation, or perceive closure as inconsequential to the overall surgical outcome. A closure that is carried out haphazardly can result in complications, which may warrant prolonged dressing changes, hospital admission, and/or additional surgical intervention. This can obviously be a significant source of distress for patients, who may suffer decreased quality of life if a chronic wound or conspicuous scar develops.

Different suturing techniques may be employed to close surgical wounds primarily [7, 8]. In order to select the best method for closure, the plastic surgeon must take into account the anatomic location, size, depth, degree of tension, patient age, comorbidities, presence of dead space, and overall tissue quality. An ideal closure should provide tension-free coaptation of the wound margins with adequate eversion of the skin edges. Eversion is defined as upward sloping of the skinedges so that they meet at a peak without any inversion. If eversion is not maximized at the time of primary closure, a depression at the site of closure can occur as the remodeling scar contracts downward. What follows are several techniques to facilitate accurate tissue approximation to maximize chances at achieving a stable, closed wound that is aesthetically acceptable to the patient.

14.5.1.1 Skin Markings and Temporary Closure

Preincisional skin marking with perpendicular hatch marks or temporary wound closure with skin staples or penetrating towel clamps can assist with precise skin edge approximation at the time of closure. In situations where nonelliptical tissue patterns will be removed, skin markings should be deferred until the excision is complete, any remaining excess skin (dog ears) has been excised, and the wound is ready for closure. In smaller wounds, a single skin hook placed at the wound apex with gentle upward traction can facilitate proper alignment of the skin edges. For large wounds under significant tension, early "tailor tacking" of the wound is advised to maximize mechanical creep and minimize desiccation and edema of the soft tissues. Once the wound edges have been temporarily opposed, buried interrupted dermal sutures are frequently placed, as detailed below.

14.5.1.2 Suturing Techniques for Primary Closure

14.5.1.2.1 Interrupted Buried Deep Dermal Closure

Any wound that is subject to static tension or contains significant dead space will benefit from the routine placement of inverted deep dermal sutures during closure. The proper technique will bring the dermis together to reduce overall wound tension, thereby serving as the strength layer of the closure. Deep dermal sutures also have the added benefit of being able to provide wound edge eversion and allow for the approximation of deeper tissues to obliterate dead space.

In contrast to the interrupted percutaneous suture, the orientation of the deep dermal suture inverts the knot within the wound bed. To do this, the needle is first passed from deep to superficial within one wound edge and then superficial to deep within the opposing wound edge, with care to achieve equal tissue purchase. Dermal thickness varies throughout the body and must be taken into account during suture placement. Anatomic areas with thicker dermis (e.g., back, scalp) necessitate a wider dermal bite that extends further from the wound edge compared to areas with thinner dermis (e.g., forearm, neck), where a narrower dermal bite is preferred. Regardless of dermal thickness, symmetric bites of each wound edge should be taken to prevent wound height discrepancies. Each bite must capture substantive tissue – a bite placed too deeply that comprises mostly subcutaneous fat risks suture pull-through and fat necrosis. Gently pulling the dermis out from underneath the skin edge with tissue forceps will allow good visualization to achieve an accurate dermal bite. In situations where the wound is small or the tissue is frail, a single skin hook may be placed just beneath the epidermis to serve as a retractor and ensure maximal dermal capture and wound eversion. If the situation arises where there is overlapping of the wound edges following suture placement, it is likely that there is asymmetric tissue capture between the two bites, and the suture should be cut out and replaced.

After placing satisfactory dermal bites within both wound edges, it is crucial to ensure that both suture ends remain on the same side of the suture loop during knot construction. Suture ends that lie on opposite sides of the suture loop will fail to invert the knot. When tightening each throw of the deep dermal knot, tension is applied perpendicular to the suture loop and parallel to the wound axis. This is noticeably different from the tension vector applied to the percutaneous interrupted suture, which is parallel to the suture loop and perpendicular to the axis of the wound. For central areas of the wound under significant tension, beginning with a granny knot followed by several square throws can be effective to achieve coaptation of the wound edges. The remaining throws can then be transitioned to alternating single-wrapped throws depending on surgeon preference.

Although 3–5 mm suture ends are typically left for an interrupted percutaneous suture to guard against knot slippage, deep dermal suture ends are cut on the knot to minimize foreign material and the risk of protrusion through the skin edges. As such, an additional throw is generally recommended to ensure knot security, especially if a monofilament suture is being used. Before concluding the deep dermal closure, applying gentle traction perpendicular to the wound edges can identify any prominent dermal gaps where additional suturing may be necessary. The surgeon should avoid placing an inordinate amount of deep dermal sutures to limit the foreign body reaction or risk of stitch abscess.

Most plastic surgeons utilize absorbable suture material (e.g., poliglecaprone 25, polyglactin 910, or polydioxanone) for deep dermal closures. While polyglactin 910 offers superior handling and knot security, its braided nature can abrade and pull through delicate tissues. In scenarios where prolonged wound tension is expected, a suture material with a prolonged absorption profile (e.g., polydioxanone) should be considered.

14.5.1.2.2 Running Subcuticular (Intradermal) Closure

The running subcuticular technique, first popularized by Halsted, allows for an expeditious closure of wounds of all sizes. This closure method is ideally suited for straight, clean wounds with symmetric, healthy edges, often in conjunction with interrupted deep dermal support. In plastic surgery, this most frequently includes breast, body contouring, and clean excisional procedures. In wounds with areas of devitalized skin edges, consideration should be given to sharply freshen the edges if closure with the subcuticular technique is planned. Subcuticular closure should be avoided in wounds that have irregular tissue edges or are at high risk for infection (e.g., dog bite injuries).

Classical teachings have portrayed the subcuticular closure as a perpendicular stitch with the exiting stitch on one wound edge entering the opposing skin edge directly across the wound. However, instead of entering the dermis directly across from the exiting bite on the opposite side, choosing an entrance site slightly more proximal can improve tissue apposition and the aesthetic result. During each bite, the dermis is stabilized with tissue forceps which apply gentle upward and outward traction to facilitate precise suture placement. Bites should be kept small to avoid puckering and gapping of the wound edges. The more downstream travel between bites, the greater is the risk of wound edge misalignment. It is important to avoid trauma to the wound edges (e.g., while using tissue forceps) as this can disrupt dermal blood supply and impair wound healing.

Although traditionally anchored by knots at both apices, knotless subcuticular closure is possible and prevents suture spitting and patient discomfort in the early postoperative period. In lieu of anchoring knots at each end of the wound, either the free ends of the suture can be secured with adhesive tape or the suture can be clipped at the level of the skin 1–2 cm from the wound apex.

Most plastic surgeons choose to perform a subcuticular closure using an absorbable monofilament suture (e.g., poliglecaprone 25), given its low frictional force and absorbable nature. Others will elect to perform subcuticular closure for short wounds with nonabsorbable suture material (e.g., polypropylene), with a scheduled removal. The nonabsorbable suture choice has the added benefit of leaving no residual foreign body as the wound continues to heal and remodel. Subcuticular sutures are commonly supplemented with surgical tape and/or skin adhesives, particularly if some degree of gapping of the edges remains.

14.5.1.2.3 Continuous Percutaneous Closure

Continuous percutaneous closure, sometimes referred to as the "whip stitch" or "running suture," is ideally suited for the closure of long linear wounds under minimal tension (Video 14.3).

This technique is advantageous in that it readily accommodates any developing edema of the wound edges during the healing process. In comparison, the dimensions of the interrupted suture loop remain clinically unchanged and may potentially constrict or cut through edematous tissue. The continuous closure also utilizes significantly less suture material and is considerably faster, particularly over larger areas. One significant drawback of the continuous percutaneous closure method is that it does not allow for good control of wound eversion or precise tissue approximation. Additionally, if the suture breaks in the early postoperative period, then the entire wound is likely to require reclosure to prevent dehiscence. Lastly, the tension of the suture material is distributed evenly throughout, precluding individualized tensioning of different areas of the wound.

The continuous percutaneous closure begins with a simple interrupted suture at one wound apex, followed by continuously looping the suture over the downstream wound edges in a spiral fashion until the wound is closed. Traditionally, the needle is passed at a 90° angle to the wound edge with each bite, resulting in a visible suture that crosses the wound edges at an approximately 65° angle. Because both epidermis and dermis are captured with each bite, interrupted deep dermal sutures may be superfluous in truly tensionless closures. In all other scenarios, prior deep dermal suturing is advised.

The distance between needle tissue skin purchase and skin exit depends on the anatomic location and closure length. Using that distance between skin purchases is usually appropriate for most linear closures.

Most surgeons choose to perform this technique with a monofilament, nonabsorbable suture, such as nylon or polypropylene. Choosing one of these suture types facilitates later removal as both have low frictional coefficients.

14.5.1.2.4 Simple Interrupted Closure

The simple interrupted closure offers several advantages over the continuous percutaneous method (Video 14.4).

In particular, the depth of the bite, the layers of tissue incorporated, and the tension on the closure can be carefully adjusted for each individual stitch. As such, the primary advantage of the simple interrupted closure technique is maximal local tissue control to allow for an accurate approximation of the skin edges. This is particularly useful for nonlinear wounds in cosmetically sensitive areas (e.g., traumatic facial injuries) where irregular wound edges require careful approximation, which can be difficult to accomplish with a continuous closure. Simple interrupted closure is also indicated in potentially contaminated wounds expected to drain and in wounds with tenuous blood supply. The disadvantages of the simple interrupted technique include its relatively time-consuming nature compared to the continuous closure method, which is magnified over large wound areas. The removal of multiple interrupted sutures is also more onerous compared to continuous percutaneous closure removal.

Performing this technique well requires careful attention to any preexisting tissue height discrepancies of the wound margins, which most often occur from asymmetric deep dermal suture placement or underlying tissue irregularity. Correction will maximize dermal apposition, thereby strengthening the final closure and improving the aesthetic result. For the wound edge that sits higher, a shallow and narrower bite is first performed. Following this, a deeper and wider bite is taken off the wound edge that sits lower. Both of these maneuvers will help depress the higher side of the wound. For wound edges that do not require height correction, perpendicular symmetric bites should be performed to maximize wound edge eversion. When approximating the wound edges with the initial throw, sufficient tension to allow touching of the wound edges is all that is required. Minimizing tension will preserve blood flow to the wound edge. Exerting excessive force on the tissue or overtightening the knot can result in ischemia or necrosis of the wound edge. If wound edge coaptation is met with significant wound tension, then consideration should be given to the placement of deep dermal sutures. The knot of the simple interrupted closure should be positioned symmetrically off the wound margin; doing so can also improve wound eversion and prevents irritation of the epithelializing edges. The number of throws placed should be commensurate with the selected suture material. Upon the completion of knot construction, suture ends should be cut approximately 3–5 mm long for a smaller-caliber suture (#4–0 and smaller) to prevent knot failure from slippage. The ears should be left longer (up to 10 mm) for larger-caliber suture material (#3–0 and larger). As a general rule, the length of suture ends should be cut short enough so that they do not interfere during the construction of adjacent knots.

Videos 14.5 and 14.6 present demonstrations of vertical and horizontal mattress sutures, both of which are interrupted sutures – requiring four purchases of the skin envelope to provide precise coaption of the wound edges.

Both absorbable and nonabsorbable suture materials may be used for the simple interrupted closure, depending on the anatomic location, patient age, wound tension, and tissue quality. Traumatic facial lacerations in adults are generally repaired with nonabsorbable monofilament sutures (e.g., nylon, polypropylene). When deep dermal sutures are in place to eliminate surface tension, the smallest-caliber suture material should be used to minimize the risk of track marks, particularly in the head and neck areas.

14.6 Skin Adhesives

Cyanoacrylate skin adhesives were introduced over 60 years ago and touted for their speed and ease of application for everything from minor cuts to small excisional procedures [9]. However, local inflammation from toxic breakdown products, modest tensile strengths, and uncertain cosmetic outcomes limited the widespread adoption of initial cyanoacrylates. The subsequent modification of the alkyl side chain generated newer, less toxic formulations, including 2-octyl-cyanoacrylate and N-butyl-2-cyanoacrylate, which also demonstrated more robust breaking strengths. 2-Octyl-cyanoacrylate, commonly known as Dermabond (Ethicon, Inc., Somerville, N.J.), is the newest cyanoacrylate technology to receive approval by the Food and Drug Administration (FDA) for use as a topical skin adhesive. With an improved side-effect profile and tensile strength, many surgeons have since utilized Dermabond and other cyanoacrylate derivatives in a variety of closure settings. By providing a pliable, waterproof dressing that serves as an antimicrobial barrier, the early removal of protective outer dressings is permitted; this, in turn, enables the patient to safely shower over the operative site(s).

While many plastic surgeons utilize skin adhesives as adjuncts to subcuticular closure, some will opt to use them in lieu of subcuticular or interrupted percutaneous suturing when surface tension is minimal. The latter has been the case in the emergency room setting, where Dermabond use in select clean lacerations in the pediatric population offers the possibility of closure without the need for local anesthetic injection or intravenous sedation. Given that early clinical studies equated the tensile strength of Dermabond to that of 5–0 suture, it is advisable to supplement any wound under more-than-minimal tension with a deep dermal closure layer prior to Dermabond application. However, newer products, such as Dermabond Prineo (Ethicon, Inc., Somerville, N.J.), that utilize a polyester mesh with cyanoacrylate overlay report holding strengths equivalent to that of 3–0 Monocryl.

Skin adhesives are only appropriate to close surgically created or clean wounds. Wounds at risk for developing an infection, particularly animal or human bites, should not be closed with skin adhesive. Prior to the application of skin adhesive, the wound should be clean and dry. Wounds that are amenable to deep dermal suturing should undergo suture placement to maximize wound eversion and eliminate any underlying dead space. For those full-thickness lacerations under minimal tension, it is possible to achieve wound edge eversion with Dermabond use alone.

Tissue forceps may be used to gently evert and coapt skin edges during application. Precise skin apposition must be obtained prior to application to prevent subcutaneous infiltration. The adhesive should be applied in a thin layer to prevent running and spreading to unintended sites, although this has become less frequent with the advent of the new high-viscosity formulations. Following application, patients typically do not require any further dressing. With regular daily bathing habits, Dermabond begins to slough off after an average of 5–7 days. Topical antibacterial ointments and submerging the wounds underwater should both be avoided as they can loosen or dislodge the skin adhesive.

There have been some reports of cyanoacrylate-associated contact dermatitis manifesting as nonpainful, pruritic rash. This may often be confused with postoperative cellulitis and can trigger office visits and patient phone calls. Treatment consists of the removal of the tissue adhesive and consideration of short-term use of low-potency topical steroids (e.g., hydrocortisone). Application of cyanoacrylates to open wounds or incompletely closed surgical incisions should be avoided to minimize the risk of immune sensitization.

References

1. Moy RL, Waldman B, Hein DW. A review of sutures and suturing techniques. J Dermatol Surg Oncol. 1992;18(9):785–95. https://doi.org/10.1111/j.1524-4725.1992.tb03036.x.
2. Bennett RG. Selection of wound closure materials. J Am Acad Dermatol. 1988;18(4 Pt 1):619–37. https://doi.org/10.1016/s0190-9622(88)70083-3.
3. Edlich RF, Gubler K, Wallis AG, Clark JJ, Dahlstrom JJ, Long WB 3rd. Scientific basis for the selection of skin closure techniques. J Environ Pathol Toxicol Oncol. 2010;29(4):363–72. https://doi.org/10.1615/jenvironpatholtoxicoloncol.v29.i4.70.
4. Wound Closure Manual. 2007. Ethicon.
5. Herrmann JB. Tensile strength and knot security of surgical suture materials. Am Surg. 1971;37:209–17.
6. Edlich RF, Long WB. Surgical knot tying manual. Norwalk, CT: Covidien; 2008.
7. Miller CJ, Antunes MB, Sobanko JF. Surgical technique for optimal outcomes: part II. Repairing tissues: suturing. J Am Acad Dermatol. 2015;72:389–402.
8. Jenkins LE, Davis LS. Comprehensive review of tissue adhesives. Dermatol Surg. 2018;44:1367–72.
9. James JD, Wu MM, Batra EK, Rodeheaver GT, Edlich RF. Technical considerations in manual and instrument tying techniques. J Emerg Med. 1992;10(4):469–80.

Chapter 15
Surgical Dressings

Frankie Wong, Michael Yaremchuk, Lisa Gfrerer, and Olivia Abbate Ford

15.1 Passive Dressings

Passive Dressings are categorized as primary, secondary, and tertiary depending on their distance from the surface of the wound [1].

15.1.1 Primary Dressings

A primary dressing is applied directly to the wound surface. Primary dressings protect from bacterial contamination until healing allows the closed incision to be impermeable to microorganisms. It functions as a nonadherent interface between the wound and a secondary dressing. It prevents the secondary dressing from being adherent to the wound surface and causing trauma upon removal. Xeroform

Illustrations by Ryoko Hamaguchi, MD, and Kip Carter

F. Wong
Harvard Mass General Brigham Plastic Surgery Residency Program, Boston, MA, USA

M. Yaremchuk (✉)
Division of Plastic Surgery, Massachusetts General Hospital, and The Boston Center for Ambulatory Surgery, Inc., Boston, MA, USA
e-mail: dr.y@dryaremchuk.com

L. Gfrerer · O. A. Ford
Harvard Plastic Surgery Residency Program, Boston, MA, USA

© The Author(s), under exclusive license to Springer Nature Switzerland AG 2023
M. Yaremchuk et al. (eds.), *Expertise in the Operating Room*,
https://doi.org/10.1007/978-3-031-30835-2_15

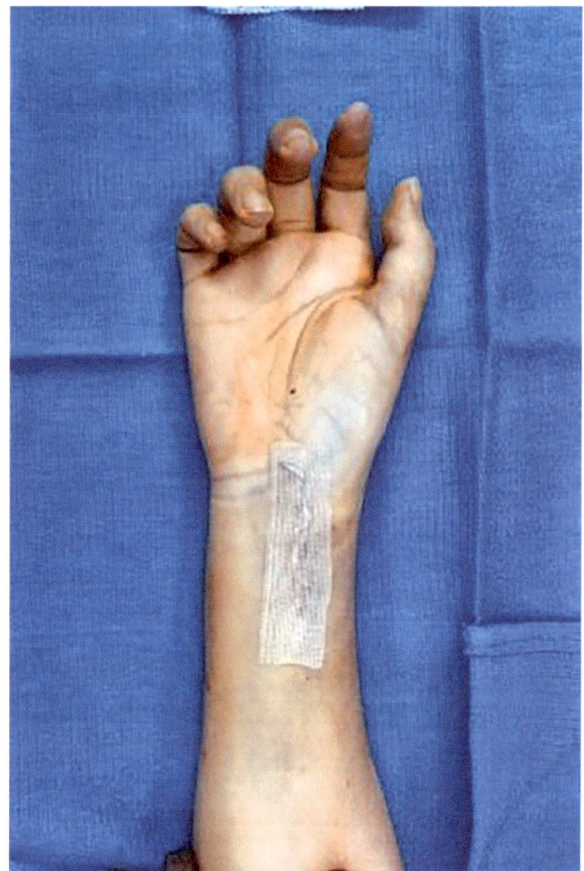

Fig. 15.1 Adaptic is functioning as the primary dressing that is part of the dressing'. for the open reduction and internal fixation (ORIF) of a distal radius fracture

petrolatum gauze is a fine mesh gauze occlusive dressing impregnated with petrolatum and 3% Xeroform (bismuth tribromophenate) ideal for the use of a surgically created wound. Another commonly used primary dressing is Adaptic (Fig. 15.1).

15.1.2 Secondary Dressings

A secondary dressing covers the primary dressing and therefore does not contact the wound. These dressings are usually made of cotton material, which absorbs exudate from the wound. They are often placed to pad and protect the wound from environmental trauma (Fig. 15.2).

Fig. 15.2 Cotton gauze is used as the secondary dressing after ORIF of a distal radius fracture

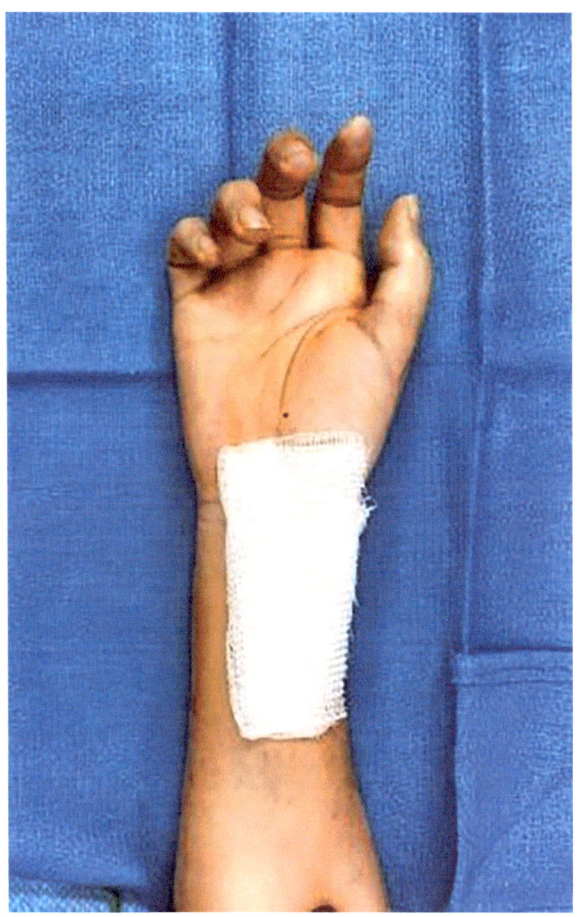

15.1.3 Tertiary Dressings

Tertiary dressings, also referred to as bandages, support primary and secondary dressings and immobilize the wound to optimize healing (Fig. 15.3).

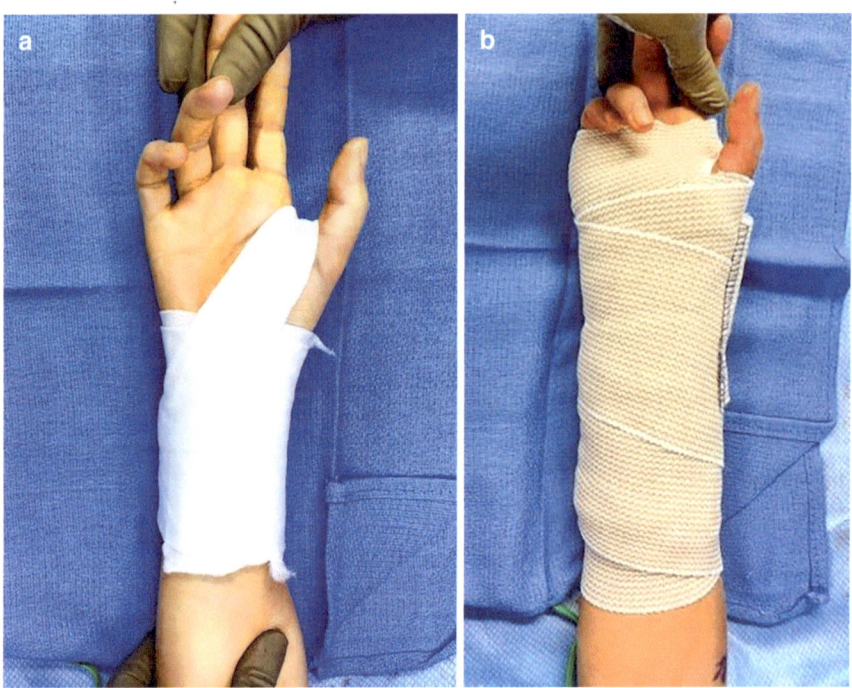

Fig. 15.3 A plaster splint secured with an ACE wrap is used as the tertiary dressing after ORIF of a distal radius fracture. (**a**) A plaster splint is placed as part of the tertiary dressing. (**b**) An ACE wrap secures the plaster cast as part of the tertiary dressing

15.2 Interactive Dressings

Interactive dressings are used to treat contaminated wounds. Contaminated wounds are classified as Class III and Class IV [2]. Class III wounds are wounds made during an operation in which major breaks in sterile technique or gross spillage from the gastrointestinal (GI) tract occurred. Class IV wounds are infected wounds with retained devitalized tissue. Contaminated and dirty/infected wounds are typically not closed primarily. Their dressings require drainage and debridement of contaminants until closure is safe.

Interactive dressings help control the microenvironment by combining with or controlling the exudate, debriding the wound, or stimulating activity in the healing cascade to speed the healing process.

There are several classes of interactive dressings, which are classified by their function depending on the amount of wound exudate. Absorbent interactive dressings include hydrocolloid, foam, alginate, hydrofiber, hydroactive, and hydrogel materials. The multiplicity of these material components, mechanisms, applications, and clinical use precludes their inclusion in this text. Rather, the authors have included the most frequently used surgical interactive dressings. The "wet-to-dry" is a long-used dressing effective in wound debridement. The more recently developed negative pressure wound therapy (NPWT), also referred to as vacuum-assisted closure (VAC), removes excess fluids as well as stimulates granulation tissue and wound contraction.

15.2.1 Wet-to-Dry Dressings

The most commonly used dressing for dirty wounds with devitalized tissue at the wound base is a "wet-to-dry" dressing. This type of dressing is used to mechanically debride open wounds [3]. Normal saline-moistened woven gauze sponges are placed directly on the wound surface. After drying, the gauze fibers adhere to devitalized tissue. Removal of the dressings mechanically debrides the attached materials. These dressings are continued until the healing by secondary intention process controls contamination to allow a delayed closure to be appropriate.

15.3 Negative Pressure Wound Therapy (NPWT)

Argenta and Morykwas developed negative pressure wound therapy (NPWT), also referred to as vacuum-assisted closure (VAC) therapy, in the 1990s [4, 5]. This modality entails placing an open-cell foam dressing into the wound cavity and applying a controlled subatmospheric pressure, which removes excess fluids and stimulates granulation tissue and wound contraction to allow the closure of wounds through secondary intention healing [6–8].

15.3.1 Basic Components

The basic components of an NPWT system are shown in Fig. 15.4 and include the following:

1. *Foam sponge:* a porous interface that allows fluids to pass through the dressing. Black-colored sponges are used for most wounds. White-colored sponges are used for less substantial wound surfaces or when placed near more fragile internal structures.
2. *Semiocclusive dressing*: dressing that allows for the sealing of the wound and keeping the wound moist throughout the duration of the therapy.
3. *Fluid collection system*: includes motor, power system, fluid collection reservoir, and vacuum device that generates negative pressure via a drainage port connected to the wound.
4. *Tubing*: includes a system for transferring fluid and air from the wound to the collection system.

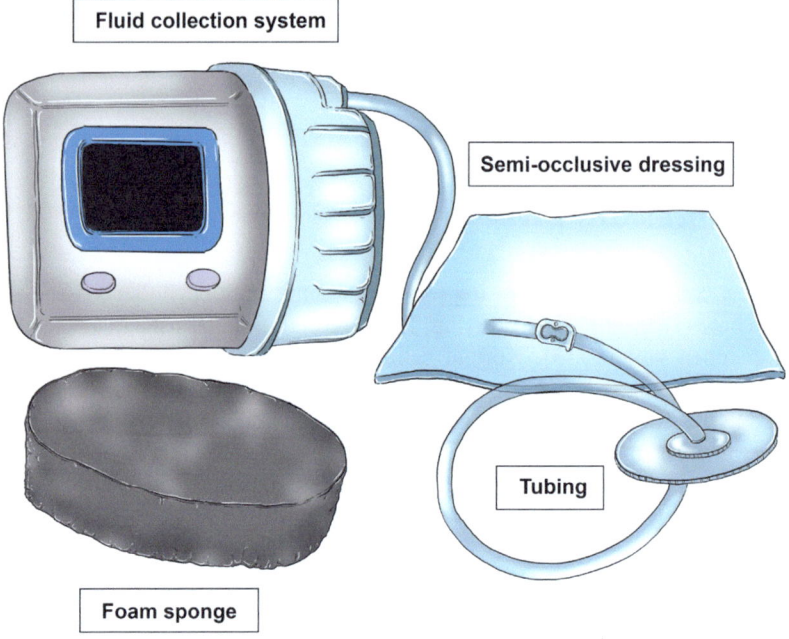

Fig. 15.4 Basic components of an NPWT system includes a foam sponge, fluid collection system, semiocclusive dressing, and tubing system

15.3.2 Mechanism of Actions of NPWT

NPWT impacts wound healing via three separate mechanisms: (1) macrostrain, (2) microstrain, and (3) fluid removal from the wound (Fig. 15.5).

15.3.2.1 Macrostrain

Macrostrain refers to the physical collapse of the wound, which is the direct result of the negative pressure applied to draw the wound edges together. The sponge system also maintains a moist and warm environment to help facilitate this process.

15.3.2.2 Microstrain

Microstrain refers to the mechanical transformation that occurs on the microscopic level when negative pressure is applied. This pressure provides stress to the cytoskeleton on a cellular level, leading to the promotion of granulation tissue formation and microvascular angiogenesis.

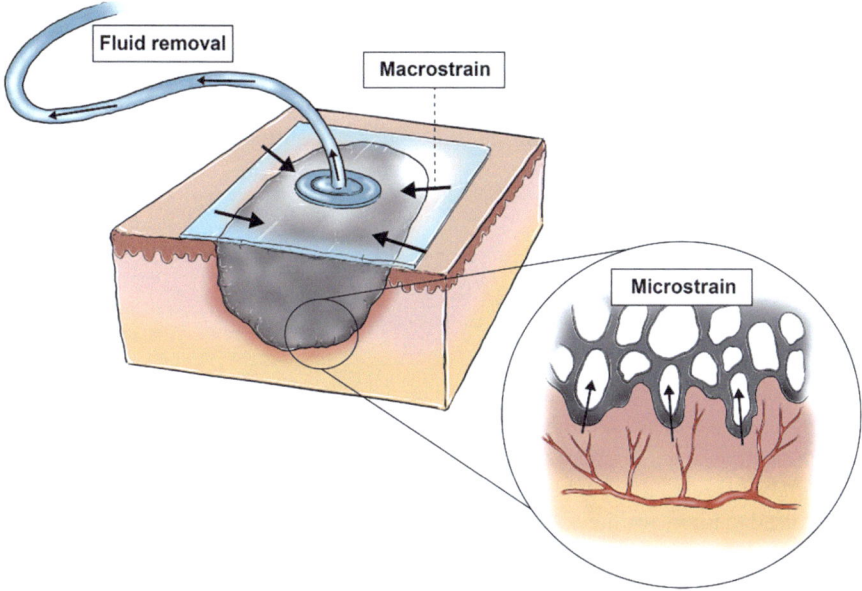

Fig. 15.5 NPWT promotes wound healing via fluid removal, microstrain, and macrostrain effects

15.3.3 Fluid Removal from the Wound

The porous structures of sponges allow fluids to be removed throughout therapy sessions. This promotes the circulation of fluid and removes exudates from leaky blood vessels and lymphatic channels into the vacuum system. This lowers the tension in the extracellular space, allowing a more optimal condition for cellular proliferation and, ultimately, wound healing.

15.3.4 Indications for NPWT

NPWT has been shown to be useful to treat diverse wounds in different anatomic locations. Common conditions for NPWT include dehisced surgical wounds, complex and larger acute wounds, pressure wounds, poorly healing diabetic and neuropathic ulcers, chronic open wounds, and after skin graft or dermal scaffold (i.e., Integra®) procedures [9–11].

15.3.5 Contraindications to NPWT

NPWT is contraindicated for the following:

1. Exposed solid organs or neurovascular structures.
2. Wounds that are grossly infected (instillation NPWT, described below, is designed for infected wounds and can sometimes be used in infected tissues).
3. Malignancy due to the theoretical promotion of angiogenesis and the proliferation of malignant cells secondary to negative pressure and its effect on the cellular cytoskeleton.

15.3.6 NPWT Application (Fig. 15.6)

1. *Wound Preparation*
   Eschar or fibrinous exudate should be debrided to healthy, punctate bleeding tissue. Hemostasis should be achieved through suture ligation, silver nitrate application, manual pressure, or a combination of the above. The wound should then be irrigated thoroughly. When the silver sponge is used, sterile water should be used to allow for the activation of silver ions. For wounds with friable tissues, or when being used after skin grafting, a layer of nonadherent dressing (e.g., Xeroform or Adaptic) should be applied prior to sponge application.
2. *Periwound Preparation*
   For wounds with increasing moisture, a degreasing agent (i.e., hydrogen peroxide or alcohol) can be used to clean and dry the wound. Then a skin preparation agent (i.e., Mastisol) can then be applied to the surrounding skin to improve the adherence of the semiocclusive agent to the periwound surface.
3. *Sponge Customization*
   The width, length, and depth of the wound are measured, and a sponge that matches the dimensions is then cut accordingly. It is important to not pack too much sponge material into the wound. The periwound surrounding the skin should not be included when designing the sponge's shape as applied pressure can cause damage to the soft tissue and skin. As the wound heals, the sponge size needed to fill the wound should decrease as well, indicating a healing wound.
4. *Sponge and Adhesive Application*
   After the appropriate sponge is tailored and crafted, the sponge can be placed into the wound, followed by the application of the included adhesive tape. This secures

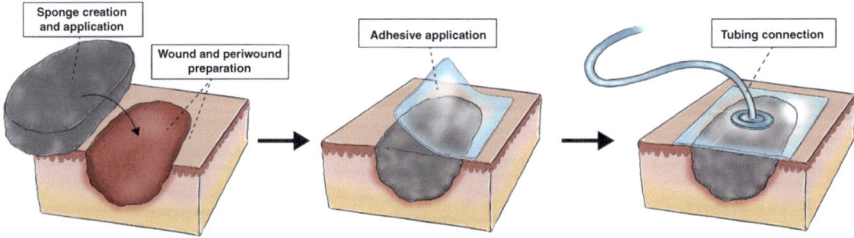

Fig. 15.6 Proper application of NPWT includes customization of sponge to fit the size of the wound, application of adhesive to secure the sponge, and connecting the tubing system

the sponge in place in the wound bed. A 2 × 2 cm^2 window can then be created by cutting the semipermeable adhesive to allow proper suction once the suction pad and tubing are connected to the negative pressure therapy device. The device can then be checked for leakage. Ideally, VAC sponges should be changed every 48 to 72 h.

5. *Instillation (Only in Indicated Wounds)*

    For the instillation system, the therapy unit will need to be programmed prior to the initiation of therapy [12, 13]. First, the fill assist function can be used to help monitor the initial wound fill to determine the correct instill volume. Then a soak interval can be set to determine the duration of time for the instillation cycle. Next, the therapy time can be set to determine the overall length of time of the cycle.

15.3.6.1 NPWT Pressure Setting

Pressure ranges from −50 to −150 mmHg and is titrated based on clinical observation of the wound after application of the NPWT system. This can then be set to either intermittent or, most often, continuous pressure. Indications for increasing the pressure setting include excessive drainage, wounds with a large volume, and difficulty maintaining a seal, especially within a tunneled wound.

Indications for decreasing the pressure setting include excessive granulation growth and excessive pressure or pain.

15.3.6.2 NPWT Removal

VAC sponges should be changed every 48 to 72 h. For patients experiencing extensive amounts of pain with sponge changes, local anesthetics can be first infused through the tubing prior to removal. After infusion, the tubing should be clamped to allow installation to occur prior to removal. For all sponge changes and removals, the suction tubing should be clamped to temporarily suspend treatment. Next, the semipermeable adhesive should be removed. An adhesive remover solution can also be used to facilitate removal to decrease skin irritation. Sponges should then be removed carefully from the wound bed to avoid excess trauma to tissue or deeper structures. If needed, normal saline can be applied intermittently to soften the interface between the sponge and the wound. Since the sponges are not bioabsorbable, it is important to remove all sponges.

15.3.7 *Potential Complications*

Inadequacies in wound preparation predispose to complications from NPWT therapy.

Bleeding may occur from inadequate hemostasis during debridement or may result from pressure-induced mechanical damage to underlying vascular structures, grafts, or organs.

Infection may occur after inadequate debridement prior to sponge placement. Dirty or contaminated wounds require frequent wound assessment and sponge replacement [14].

Retained sponges are more likely to happen in wounds with a tunneled component.

15.3.8 Troubleshooting

Leaks are the most common types of issues that prevent effective treatment. A small air leak is very common and can almost always be attributed to inadequate sealing of the sponge by the semipermeable adhesive dressing. This is commonly due to irregular body contours surrounding the wound. To prevent these leaks, the semipermeable adhesive dressing should not be stretched and should be placed in a manner that encompasses the entire wound edge. These leaks can be fixed by identifying the area of the inadequate seal. If a small leak is present, this will often present as a high pitch sound arising from the periphery of the semipermeable dressing. An additional adhesive dressing can then be applied to reinforce these areas of leaks. If a larger leak is present, manual pressure might need to be applied to the perisponge surface to determine the location of the leak. Damage or breaks in the tubing system itself and/or the suction canister interface should be considered when troubleshooting for leaks.

Suction blockage during NPWT therapy may result from external pressure on the suction tubing itself or from blood clots within the suction tubing, the sponge, or the wound. Clots in the suction tubing can be dislodged by infusing a small amount of saline into the tubing. Clots in the wound or sponge itself require sponge replacement. Clots or blockages in the suction canister require canister replacement.

15.3.9 Difficult Scenarios

15.3.9.1 Y Technique

The Y technique allows one VAC therapy unit to treat multiple adjacent wounds simultaneously. The Y connector allows an equal amount of pressure to apply to each of the wounds (Fig. 15.7).

15.3.9.2 Bridging Technique

The bridging technique is similar to the Y technique and allows two wounds to be treated with a single VAC therapy [15]. To utilize this technique, a strip of foam sponge needs to be crafted. The length of the strip will be based on the distance

Fig. 15.7 Y connector

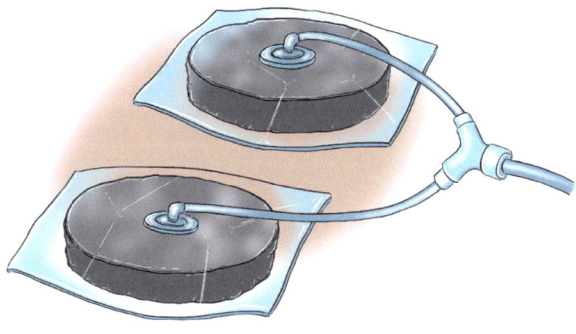

Fig. 15.8 Bridging technique

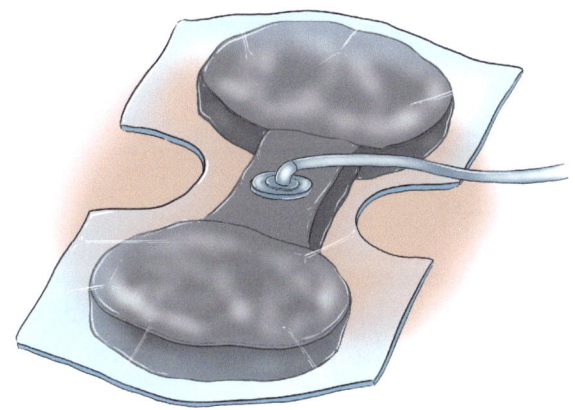

between the wound and the ideal placement of the suction pad and tubing or the distance between the two wounds to be bridged. Skin protectant dressing should then be applied to the skin that the bridge will cover. The strip of sponge is then placed and should be secured with a semipermeable adhesive dressing in the usual fashion. A keyhole can then be created at the desired location where the suction pad and tubing can be placed.

The bridging technique has many applications. It can be used to place the suction pad and tubing in a more beneficial anatomic location, such as wounds on the foot, back, or flank. Bridging allows for the suction tubing exit site, which prevents pressure injuries or maintains adequate suction. Bridging can be used to connect wounds when a Y connector is not available or indicated (Fig. 15.8).

15.3.9.3 Fecal Incontinence

Fecal incontinence poses a significant risk for wound contamination, especially with regard to perineal and sacral wounds. The moisture in this area creates a difficult area to maintain a sufficient wound seal. To prevent contamination, a protective periwound border can be applied to minimize breakdown and moisture. For the acutely ill patient, or insensate patient, a fecal collection system can also be used to help divert potential fecal contamination. Nevertheless, sponges should be changed at more frequent intervals to assess for possible wound contamination.

15.3.9.4 Tunneling

Most commonly, wound tunneling occurs due to wound infection resulting in subcutaneous tissue destruction. Tunnels are also seen in pressure wounds and in wounds where poor wound-packing techniques have been used. The tissue quality of tunneled wounds is often more friable as these areas are likely to be in an extended inflammatory phase. For these wounds, a white foam sponge should be placed into the tunnel to decrease tissue damage. The sponge can then be connected to a regular black polyurethane sponge near the surface of the wound to allow for proper wound sealing.

References

1. Sood A, Granick MS, Tomaselli NL. Wound dressings and comparative effectiveness data. Adv Wound Care (New Rochelle). 2014;3(8):511–29. https://doi.org/10.1089/wound.2012.0401. PMID: 25126472; PMCID: PMC4121107.
2. Onyekwelu I, Yakkanti R, Protzer L, Pinkston CM, Tucker C, Seligson D. Surgical wound classification and surgical site infections in the orthopaedic patient. J Am Acad Orthop Surg Glob Res Rev. 2017;1(3):e022. https://doi.org/10.5435/JAAOSGlobal-D-17-00022. PMID: 30211353; PMCID: PMC6132296.
3. Fleck CA. Why "wet to dry"? J Am Col Certif Wound Spec. 2009;1(4):109–13.
4. Winter GD. Formation of the scab and the rate of epithelization of superficial wounds in the skin of the young domestic pig. Nature. 1962;193:293–4. https://doi.org/10.1038/193293a0. PMID: 14007593.
5. Argenta LC, Morykwas MJ. Vacuum-assisted closure: a new method for wound control and treatment: clinical experience. Ann Plast Surg. 1997;38(6):563–76; discussion 577. PMID: 9188971.
6. Goss SG, Schwartz JA, Facchin F, Avdagic E, Gendics C, Lantis JC 2nd. Negative pressure wound therapy with instillation (NPWTi) better reduces post-debridement bioburden in chronically infected lower extremity wounds than NPWT alone. J Am Coll Clin Wound Spec. 2014;4(4):74–80. https://doi.org/10.1016/j.jccw.2014.02.001. PMID: 26199877; PMCID: PMC4495738.
7. Panayi A, Leavitt T, Orgill D. Evidence based review of negative pressure wound therapy. World J Dermatol. 2017;6:1–16. https://doi.org/10.5314/wjd.v6.i1.1.
8. Anghel EL, Kim PJ. Negative-pressure wound therapy: a comprehensive review of the evidence. Plast Reconstr Surg. 2016;138(3 Suppl):129S–37S. https://doi.org/10.1097/PRS.0000000000002645. PMID: 27556753.
9. Peterkar KS, Dhanraj P, Kingsly PM, Sreekar H, Lakshmanarao A, Lamba S, Shetty R, Zachariah JR. A prospective randomized controlled trial comparing negative pressure dressing and conventional dressing methods on split-thickness skin grafts in burned patients. Burns. 2011;37(6):926–9. https://doi.org/10.1016/j.burns.2011.05.013. Epub 2011 Jul 1. PMID: 21723044.

10. Maduba CC, Nnadozie UU, Modekwe VI, Onah II. Split skin graft take in leg ulcers: conventional dressing versus locally adapted negative pressure dressing. J Surg Res. 2020;251:296–302. https://doi.org/10.1016/j.jss.2020.01.029. Epub 2020 Mar 18. PMID: 32199338.
11. Yin Y, Zhang R, Li S, Guo J, Hou Z, Zhang Y. Negative-pressure therapy versus conventional therapy on split-thickness skin graft: a systematic review and meta-analysis. Int J Surg. 2018;50:43–8. https://doi.org/10.1016/j.ijsu.2017.12.020. Epub 2017 Dec 29. PMID: 29292216.
12. Gupta S, Gabriel A, Lantis J, Téot L. Clinical recommendations and practical guide for negative pressure wound therapy with instillation. Int Wound J. 2016;13(2):159–74. https://doi.org/10.1111/iwj.12452. Epub 2015 May 23. PMID: 26011379; PMCID: PMC7949544.
13. Gabriel A, Shores J, Heinrich C, Baqai W, Kalina S, Sogioka N, Gupta S. Negative pressure wound therapy with instillation: a pilot study describing a new method for treating infected wounds. Int Wound J. 2008;5(3):399–413. https://doi.org/10.1111/j.1742-481X.2007.00423.x. PMID: 18593390; PMCID: PMC7951189.
14. Prevention. CoDCa. Surgical site infection (SSI) Event national healthcare safety network; 2019. https://www.cdc.gov/nhsn/pdfs/pscmanual/9pscssicurrent.pdf.
15. Nather A, Hong NY, Lin WK, Sakharam JA. Effectiveness of bridge V.A.C. dressings in the treatment of diabetic foot ulcers. Diabet Foot Ankle. 2011;2011:2. https://doi.org/10.3402/dfa.v2i0.5893.

Index

A
A-alpha fibers, 106
A-beta fibers, 106
Absorbable sutures, 89, 90, 91
Active drains
    antibiotics, 131
    design, 130, 131
    function, 129, 130
    indications, 129
    removal of, 131
    skin exit and stabilization, 131
A-delta fibers, 106
Adson-Brown forceps, 72
Adson forceps, 71
A-gamma fibers, 106
Airway assessment, 16
Allergic reaction, 108
Allis forceps, 76
Amine, 104
Anesthesiologist's and nursing team
    airway assessment, 16
    anesthesia specific history form, 14
    CRA, 15
    data-driven pathways, 9
    emergency equipment/planning for crisis/contingency, 17
    medications, 17
    patient physical examination, 14, 15
    perioperative/circulator nurse, 18
    preference cards, 19
    red flag diagnosis, 10–13
    risk management, 10
    standard preparation, 17
    surgical and CRA, 16
    transfusion, need for, 18

Angiotensin converting enzyme inhibitors (ACEI), 11, 14
Angiotensin receptor blockers (ARB), 11, 14
Anticoagulants, 11
Antigenic para-aminobenzoic acid, 105
Army-Navy retractor, 78
Aspirin-like drugs, 6, 7
Association of periOperative Registered Nurses (AORN), 61

B
Babcock forceps, 76
Barbed suture, 94
Bard Parker scalpel, 66
Beta-blockers, 11
B fibers, 106
Bioburden, 55
Bipolar electrosurgery, 117, 118
Blend-cut function, 114
Blood pressure, 12
Blood transfusion, 18
Bonney forceps, 73
Bookwalter retractor, 81
Bridging technique, 159

C
Cardiac implantable electronic devices (CIED), 117
Cardiac risk assessment (CRA), 15, 16
Cardiovascular toxicity, 107

Centers for Disease Control and Prevention (CDC), 131
Central Nervous System (CNS) toxicity, 107
C fibers, 106
Chlorhexidine solutions (Chloraprep), 41
Coagulation, 114
Cocaine intoxication, 11
Coefficient of friction, 87
Collagen-derived sutures, 90
Conventional cutting needle, 98
Crile (Snap forceps), 77

D
DeBakey forceps, 74
Dever retractor, 80
Digital ischemia, 108
Drains
  active (suction)
    antibiotics, 131
    design, 130, 131
    function, 129, 130
    indications, 129
    removal of, 131
    skin exit and stabilization, 131
  passive
    design, 132, 133
    indications, 132
    positioning, 133
    removal of, 133
    skin immobilization, 133
Dressings
  interactive
    Class III and IV wounds, 152
    wet-to-dry, 153
  NPWT, 153
    application, 156, 157
    basic components, 153, 154
    bridging technique, 158, 159
    contraindications, 155, 156
    fecal incontinence, 159
    fluid removal from wound, 155
    indications, 155
    mechanism of actions, 154
    potential complications, 157
    troubleshooting, 158
    wound tunneling, 160
    Y technique, 158
  passive
    primary, 149
    secondary, 150
    tertiary, 151
Duration of Action (DOA), 104, 105

E
Elasticity, 87
Electrical current, 117
Electrocautery
  bipolar electrosurgery, 117, 118
    intraoperative use, 118
  monopolar, 112
    intraoperative use of, 113
    modes of operation, 112–114
  monopolar safety
    burn injury, 115
    fire, 114, 115
    jewelry, 115, 116
    pacemakers and ICD interference, 117
Electrosurgical unit (ESU), 45, 46, 111, 112, 114–117
Epinephrine, 106
Ergonomics
  effective lighting, 52
  instrument selection and passing, 54, 55
  operating table, 51
  operative personnel assist, 53
  operative site
    instruments, 55
    the patient, 55
  retraction, 53
  team positioning, 52
Esters, 105

F
Fire prevention, 58
Fires, in operating room
  airway and non-airway fires, 60, 61
  fuel, 58, 60
  ignition source, 58, 59
  oxidizer, 57, 59
  resources, 61
  specific guidelines for using laser, 60
Flash sterilization, 29
Forearm tourniquet, 122
Frazier suctioning, 82
Fuel, 58

G
Gastroesophageal reflux, 13
Gelpi retractor, 80

H
Heart rate, 12
Hegar needle holder, 83

Hemoglobin, 18
Hemostasis, 55, 106
Hook retractor, 79

I
Ignition source, 58
Implantable cardioverter-defibrillator (ICD), 117
Installation system, 157
Instruments, *see* Surgical instruments
Intermittent pneumatic compression (IPC), 46
Iodine povacrylex with isopropyl alcohol, 41
Iris forceps, 72
Iris scissors, 70

J
Jacobson/mosquito forcep, 76

K
Kelly forceps, 77
Knot security, 87
Kocher design forceps, 77

L
Light emitting diodes (LED), 52
Limb occlusion pressure (LOP), 123
Lipid emulsion therapy, 108
Lipid solubility, 105
Local anesthetics
   DOA, 104, 105
   dosing, 106
   management of suspected toxicity, 108
   mechanism of action, 103
   molecular structure, 104
      time for onset, 104
   nerve fibers and their sequence of blockade, 105, 106
   potency, 105
   safety and toxicity, 107, 108
   types of, 105
   vasoconstrictors and hemostasis, 106
Logistics, *see* Ergonomics
Lonestar retractor system, 81

M
Macrostrain, 154

Mayo scissors, 68
Mechanism of action, 103
Memory, 86
Metabolic equivalents (METs), 15
Methemoglobinemia toxicity, 108
Metzenbaum (Metz) scissors, 69, 70
Microstrain, 154
Mixter (right angle forceps), 77
Monofilament suture, 88
Monopolar electrocautery (Bovie), 112–114
Multifilament sutures, 88

N
Nasotracheal tube immobilization, 36
Needles
   needle curvatures, 96, 97
   point
      blunt point, 99
      conventional cutting, 97
      holders, 99, 100
      reverse cutting, 98
      taper tip, 98
   sutures attachment, eye/swage, 95
Negative pressure wound therapy (NPWT), 153
   application
      installation system, 157
      periwound preparation, 156
      sponge and adhesive application, 156
      sponge customization, 156
      wound preparation, 156
   basic components, 153, 154
   bridging technique, 158, 159
   contraindications, 155, 156
   fecal incontinence, 159
   fluid removal from wound, 155
   indications, 155
   mechanism of actions, 154
   potential complications, 157
   troubleshooting, 158
   wound tunneling, 160
   Y technique, 158
Nonabsorbable suture, 89, 91, 93
Nonpneumatic tourniquets, 122

O
Obstructive sleep apnea (OSA), 13
Open reduction and internal fixation (ORIF), 150
Operating room (OR) fires, 57–61

Operating room preparation
    anesthesiologist's and nursing team
        airway assessment, 16
        anesthesia specific history form, 14
        CRA, 15
        data-driven pathways, 9
        emergency equipment/planning for crisis/contingency, 17
        medications, 17
        patient physical examination, 14, 15
        perioperative/circulator nurse, 18
        preference cards, 19
        red flag diagnosis, 10–13
        risk management, 10
        standard preparation, 17
        surgical and CRA, 16
        transfusion, need for, 18
    surgeon's preparation
        aspirin-like drugs, 6, 7
        consent for surgery, 3
        fundamental responsibility, 3, 4
        patient preoperative timeline, 4–6
Opioid use disorder (OUD), 11
Oxidizers, 58
Oxygen delivery, 59

P
Para-chloro-meta-xylenol (PCMX), 41
Passive drains
    design, 132, 133
    indications, 132
    positioning, 133
    removal of, 133
    skin immobilization, 133
Patient positioning, 39
Patient preparation
    airway, 35
    draping, 44
    ear canal, 38
    endotracheal tube security, 36
    eye protection, 37
    intraoral and intranasal surgery, 37
    IPC devices, 46
    monopolar electrocautery, 45, 46
    nasotracheal tube security, 36
    positioning, 39, 40
    skin preparation
        debridement, 40
        solutions, 41–43
    tubing and cords, 45
Penrose drain, 133
Percutaneous coronary intervention (PCI), 12
Permanent pacemakers (PPMs), 117
Physical examination, 14, 15
Plasticity, 87
Pneumatic tourniquets, 122
Polydioxanone, 89, 92
Polypropylene, 93, 94
Potency, 105
Primary wound closure
    continuous percutaneous closure, 145
    interrupted buried deep dermal closure, 143, 144
    running subcuticular (intradermal) closure, 144, 145
    simple interrupted closure, 146
    skin marking and temporary closure, 142, 143

R
Rat Tooth forceps, 73
Red flag diagnosis, 10–13
Reverse cutting needle, 98

S
Senn retractor, 79
Skin adhesives, 147, 148
Sterilization
    operating staff
        ATTIRE, 27, 28
        avoiding hand contamination, 28
        hand drying, 29
        hand preparation/scrubbing, 28
        OR environment, 29
        surgical instruments, 29, 30
    patient
        antibiotics, 30
        intraoperative optimization, 30
        preoperative preparation, 30
Suctioning, 55
Surgeon's preparation
    aspirin-like drugs, 6, 7
    consent for surgery, 3
    fundamental responsibility, 3, 4
    patient preoperative timeline, 4–6
Surgical instruments, 29
    clamps (locking forceps), 75–78
    cutting and dissecting, 65
    forceps
        smooth, 74, 75
        toothed, 71–73
    hand-held retractors
        Army-Navy, 78

Dever, 80
hook, 79
Richardson, 80
Senn-Miller, 79
needle holder, 82
scalpels
knife handles, 67, 68
standard blades, 66, 67
scissors
iris, 70
Mayo, 68
Metzenbaum, 69, 70
tenotomy, 70
self-retaining retractors, 80, 81
simple retractors, 78
suctioning, 81, 82
Suture
absorbable
chromic gut, 89, 91
Monocryl (Poliglecaprone 25), 89, 92
plain gut, 89, 91, 92
polydioxanone, 92
Vicryl (Polyglactin 910), 89, 92
barbed suture, 94
biomechanical properties
coefficient of friction, 87
elasticity, 87
knot security, 87
memory, 86
tensile strength, 86
tissue reactivity, 88
classifications, 89
diameter, 85
monofilament, 88
multifilament, 88
nonabsorbable
nylon, 90, 93, 94
polyesters, 94
prolene (polypropylene), 93
silk, 93
physical characteristics, 89
topical skin adhesives, 95
varying sizes of, 86
Suture closure
instrument tying, 141, 142
knot construction, 138
slip and square knots, 139
knot failure, 139
primary wound closure (*see* Primary wound closure)
skin adhesives, 147, 148
surgical knot, 137, 138
two-handed knot tying, 140, 141

T
Taper ratio, 98
Taper tip needle, 99
Tenotomy scissors, 70
Tensile strength, 86
Tertiary dressings, 151
Time-tested approach, 131
Tissue forceps stabilize tissues, 70
Tonsil Schnidt forceps, 78
Tourniquet
application, 122
effects and complications, 124, 125
guidelines, 123, 124
placement, 123
use of, 121, 122
Toxicity
allergic reaction, 108
cardiovascular, 107
CNS, 107
digital ischemia, 108
methemoglobinemia, 108

U
Universal protocol, 23–26

V
Vacuum-assisted closure (VAC), 153
Vasoconstrictors, 106
Visualization, 37

W
Weitlaner retractor, 81

Y
Yankauer suctioning tool, 81

MIX
Papier aus verantwortungsvollen Quellen
Paper from responsible sources
FSC® C105338

If you have any concerns about our products,
you can contact us on
ProductSafety@springernature.com

In case Publisher is established outside the EU,
the EU authorized representative is:
**Springer Nature Customer Service Center GmbH
Europaplatz 3, 69115 Heidelberg, Germany**

Printed by Libri Plureos GmbH
in Hamburg, Germany